STERILIZATION VALIDATION & ROUTINE OPERATION HANDBOOK

STERILIZATION VALIDATION & ROUTINE OPERATION HANDBOOK
Radiation

Anne F. Booth
President
Booth Scientific, Inc.

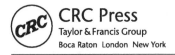

CRC Press
Taylor & Francis Group
Boca Raton London New York

CRC Press is an imprint of the
Taylor & Francis Group, an **informa** business

Sterilization Validation & Routine Operation Handbook

First published 2001 by CRC Press
Taylor & Francis Group
6000 Broken Sound Parkway NW, Suite 300
Boca Raton, FL 33487-2742

Reissued 2018 by CRC Press

A Library of Congress record exists under LC control number: 2001087245

Publisher's Note
The publisher has gone to great lengths to ensure the quality of this reprint but points out that some imperfections in the original copies may be apparent.

Disclaimer
The publisher has made every effort to trace copyright holders and welcomes correspondence from those they have been unable to contact.

ISBN 13: 978-1-138-50673-2 (hbk)
ISBN 13: 978-1-138-56193-9 (pbk)
ISBN 13: 978-0-203-71022-7 (ebk)

Visit the Taylor & Francis Web site at http://www.taylorandfrancis.com and the CRC Press Web site at http://www.crcpress.com

Main entry under title:
    Sterilization Validation & Routine Operation Handbook: Radiation

Bibliography: p. 155

Table of Contents

Acknowledgement

I would like to express my thanks to Craig Herring at Ethicon Endo-Surgery, Inc. for his technical review of this manuscript. His constructive comments and suggestions guaranteed that the most accurate and complete information available was included in this book.

Introduction

THE following handbook is intended to provide a framework for the validation and routine operation of an irradiation sterilization process. The guidance presented complies with ANSI/AAMI/ISO 11137: 1994, *Sterilization of health care product—Requirements for validation and routine control—Radiation sterilization.* Be advised that ISO 11137 is currently under revision, and revision elements known at the time of publication have been incorporated into this handbook. The standard provides a framework and should not be considered inflexible or static. This handbook defines methods to assist in the interpretation and understanding of the requirements in this standard as well as other ancillary standards and guidelines and offers practical procedures for the validation and routine monitoring of specific radiation sterilization processes. Just a reminder: medical devices should be manufactured employing a quality system complying with ISO 9001 or ISO 9002 and FDA Code of Federal Regulations 21 CFR Part 820.

CHAPTER 1

Rationale for Validating Sterilization Processes

THE basic requirement for validating manufacturing processes, of which sterilization is one, is defined in the Food and Drug Administration's Quality System Regulation 21 CFR Part 820, Sec. 820.75, "Where the results of a process cannot be fully verified by subsequent inspection and test, the process shall be validated with a high degree of assurance and approved according to established procedures. The validation activities and results, including the date and signature of the individual(s) approving the validation and where appropriate the major equipment validated, shall be documented."

While following this mandate in the validation of a sterilization process, additional assurance is obtained during the process by doing the following:

- defining and documenting the hardware and software used in the process and the operating characteristics of each piece of equipment.
- verifying the microbial kill (sterility assurance level)
- insuring by monitoring with dosimeters that the minimum sterilization dose process is delivered and is reproducible from run to run
- confirming that the routine monitoring positions and the data obtained from these locations is sufficient to control the process

In addition, the ISO 9000 series designates certain processes used in manufacturing as "special" in that the results cannot be fully verified by subsequent inspection and testing of the product. Sterilization is one of these special processes, and for this reason, it requires validation before use. The performance of the process also needs to be monitored routinely.

Be aware that exposure to a properly validated and accurately controlled sterilization process is not the only factor associated with the provision of reliable assurance that the product is sterile. Attention should also be given to several other factors including the following:

- microbiological status (bioburden) of raw materials
- resistance of the bioburden to the sterilizing agent
- control of the manufacturing environment
- packaging of the product and loading for processing
- maintenance of the equipment and dosimeters
- appropriateness of the sterilization dose

ASPECTS OF A RADIATION STERILIZATION PROGRAM

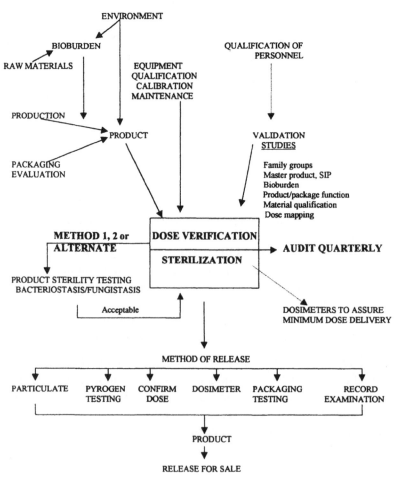

The radiation process is a physical one. It involves exposure of product to ionizing radiation in equipment specially designed to deliver gamma rays from cobalt 60 or cesium 137 or by electron or X-ray beams delivered by an electron beam accelerator. The validation process must be documented, monitored at a higher level than routine production cycles, and repeated to show consistency of operation and microbial kill. The validation will serve to define the limits of routine processing.

The entire sterilization system consists of multiple components, all of which require application of quality procedures, operator training, continuous monitoring, and failure investigation when necessary. The elements of the system are illustrated on page 2 and will be discussed at length in this Handbook. Use this handy reference to establish and maintain your radiation sterilization processes and to assess test methods that are most appropriate for your products.

CHAPTER 2

Characterization of
Radiation Processes ·

Two different types of radiation processes are used in industrial radiation processing of medical products, i.e., gamma rays and electron beams (see Figure 1). A third type, X-rays, has been shown to have microbiocidal effects, but this method is not currently available for industrial sterilization. The microbial lethality of gamma rays and electrons is accomplished by ionization; electrons are direct ionizing radiation, whereas photons are indirect ionizing radiation. The energy transferred by these radiations during the sterilization process produces chemical and/or physical changes at the molecular level resulting in chain scission, polymerization, cross-linking, sterilization, and disinfection.

PHYSICAL CHARACTERISTICS OF RADIATION

By far, the most commonly used of the three methods is gamma radiation. Gamma rays are emitted from radioactive isotope source materials, the most common being cobalt 60 (^{60}Co). Gamma rays are electromagnetic waves frequently referred to as photons. Having no electric charge or mass, photons transfer energy to materials mainly through Compton scattering collisions with atomic electrons resulting in a uniform, exponentially decreasing depth dose distribution (see Figure 2). The photons strike free electrons in the material and pass part of their energy to the electron as kinetic energy. These displaced electrons continue on their way, deflected from their original path. The scattered gamma ray carries the balance of the energy as it moves off through the material, possibly to interact again with another electron. In the place of the incident photon, there are now a number of fast electrons and photons of reduced energy that may go on to take part in

5

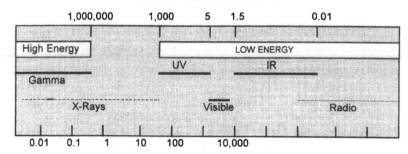

ENERGY-ELECTRON VOLTS

WAVELENGTHS - ANGSTROM UNITS (Log scale)

Figure 1 Wavelengths and energy levels of different types of electromagnetic radiation.

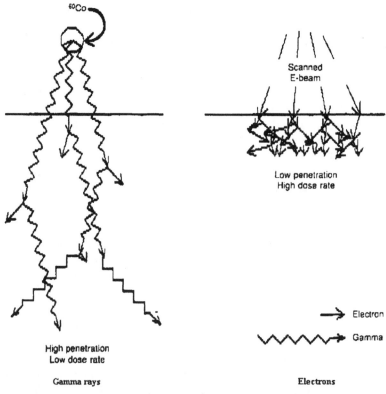

Figure 2 Penetration pattern of gamma and electron beam radiation (adapted from Bernard, 1991).

6

further reactions. It is the cascade of electrons that results in the physical and chemical changes in the material and the destruction of microorganisms. Because the probability of Compton scattering is low, the primary beam of gamma rays will penetrate long distances in material before the scattering occurs. This means that the gamma rays deposit energy over a relatively large area so that penetration is high (up to 50 cm), but the dose rate is low.

In contrast to gamma rays, electrons focused into a beam generated by a linear accelerator with beam energies of 5–10 MeV have both mass and charge, so they interact readily with other charged particles, transferring their kinetic energy to materials by numerous elastic and inelastic collisions. In fact, as soon as charged particles penetrate solid materials, they are subject to the Colomb force exerted by the atomic nuclei and are, therefore, in almost constant interaction with the material. These interactions result in many directional changes, ionizations, and radioactive processes that slow the electrons and ultimately limit their penetration to only 5 cm into material with a density of 1.0 gm/cm^{-3} using a 10 MeV beam (see Figure 2). E-beam energy is therefore deposited within materials over a short distance, making the dose rate very high (22,000 kGy/hour for a 50-kW beam) and allowing sterilization to take place in less than one minute.

The parameter measuring the energy transferred from the radiation source to the product is called the absorbed dose. The dose can be translated in terms of power requirements (i.e., intensity and energy of the beam) by taking into account the product characteristics (shape, size, and density) and the process parameters (i.e., throughput, scanning length). The penetration of gamma rays and electrons is inversely proportional to product density. The absorbed dose is the quantity of ionizing radiation energy imparted per unit mass of a specified material and is expressed as the Gray (Gy), where 1 Gy = 100 Rads or 1 kGy = 0.1 Megarad.

FACILITY DESIGN

The gamma facility radioactive source is housed in a thin rod or "pencil" about 18″ long; each one contains approximately 10,000 curies of ^{60}Co. The pencils are held in a rack that is kept in a pool of water when not in use. The number of photons emitted per second is a function of the number of curies in the source. Each curie of ^{60}Co emits 7.4×10^{10} photons per second. A typical facility will contain more than one million curies of isotope allowing large volumes of products to be treated in relatively short periods of time. When in use, the source rack is elevated out of the pool and the product to be sterilized passes around the source.

E-beam sterilization is a machine-based radiation method. The operation of an electron accelerator is similar to that of a television set, in that both employ a source of electrons focused into a beam. There are two types of electron accelerators: direct current (Dynamitron) which requires the generation of high electron potentials, and indirect accelerators (linear) which produce high electron energies by repetitive application of time-varying electromagnetic fields. Both systems are built with output beam power of 10–100 kW. Electron beams can be either vertical which facilitates conveyor loading or horizontal which facilitates two-sided irradiation (see Figure 3). A comparison of the two systems is summarized in Table 1.

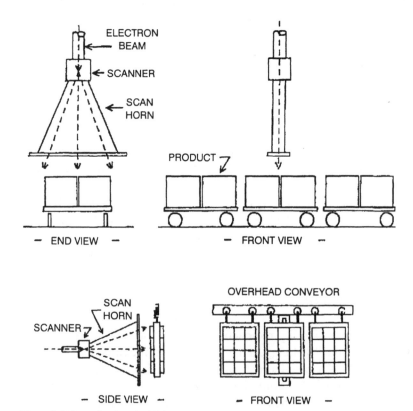

Figure 3 Schematic of vertical E-beam scan horn (top) and horizontal scan horn (bottom).

TABLE 1. Characteristics of Gamma and E-Beam Sterilization Systems (adapted from Farrell and Hemmerich, 1995).

Property	Gamma	Electron Beam
Energy spectrum	1.17 and 1.33 MeV	10 ± 1 MeV
Decay rate	12.6% per year	NA
Electrical efficiency	NA	15–35%
Useful power range	15–100 kW (1–7 MCi)	10–200 kW
Typical dose rate	1–10 kGy/hour	2–50 kGy/second

EFFECTS OF RADIATION ON MICROORGANISMS

When a population of microbial cells is irradiated, the number of living units diminishes exponentially as the dose increases, until no viable cells remain. Sterility is obtained in living organisms in two ways: directly through DNA strand rupture or through cell destruction related to chemical reactions in the organism or in its environment. Energy can be directly deposited in a bond of a macromolecule (protein, DNA, RNA) causing a rearrangement of its structure, or free radicals can be generated from the water contained within the cell. The free radicals then react with the macromolecule, altering its normal cellular metabolism which leads to loss of the reproductive capacity of the microorganism. In a nonaqueous environment, as found in the sterilization of most medical devices, the principal sterilization mechanism is ionization of cellular material altering molecular structure or spatial configuration of biologically active molecules.

The number of organisms inactivated by a given radiation dose is a statistical phenomenon. It depends on the sensitivity of the microorganism to alterations of biologically active molecules and their ability to repair the alterations. Different organisms will have different capabilities of withstanding and repairing damage. It has been shown that microorganisms are inactivated by first-order kinetics, which can be represented by a dose/survival curve (Figure 4), where the fractional survival is plotted on a semilog scale. The probability of survival can then be predicted assuming this exponential relationship. The D_{10} value for a particular organism is the dose required to reduce the population of that organism to 10% of its original level. It is determined from the linear part of the curve. Thus, irradiation of a family of organisms will give rise to a family of curves as seen in Figure 4. The choice of a sterilization dose for a particular product must be based on knowledge of the types of organisms found on or in the product. The greater

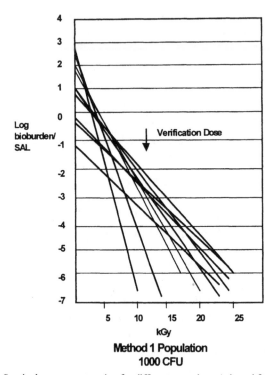

Method 1 Population
1000 CFU

Figure 4 Survival curve construction for different organisms (adapted from Phillips).

the degree of contamination, the higher the radiation dose required to achieve the desired level of inactivation. The lower the initial bioburden, the greater the likelihood that the variety of organisms will be limited to one or a few species. Mammalian cells are the most sensitive to radiation. Fungi, bacteria, and viruses have so much overlap that there is no clear order of resistance (see Table 21).

SYSTEM OPERATIONS

Gamma and E-beam systems operate in a similar fashion. Outside the irradiation source on the nonsterile side of the facility, product is loaded into carriers or totes. An automatic conveyor system then moves the loaded product into the shielded irradiation chamber past the gamma ray source or the electron beam. In order to maximize dose uniformity, the product passes the source with two opposing sides exposed. After passing through the radiation field for a specified time interval or at a specified speed, the product exits the process chamber into the sterile side of the facility, where it is held until dosimeters are read to verify that the correct radiation dose was delivered. When this is confirmed, the product is released for shipment; no sterility test is required.

Gamma irradiation can take place in a batch [Figure 5(b)] or continuous [Figure 5(a)] process. In the batch-type process, the products run by themselves or only with other products of a similar density, so product mixing is of little concern. Consequently, there is usually no problem accommodating products with greatly different process specifications in any sequence. In a continuous-type process, the products must fit into a continuous but variable string of products

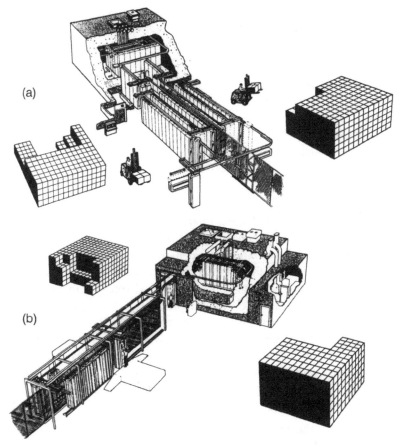

Figure 5 (a) Continuous gamma irradiator and (b) batch-carrier gamma irradiator. Both courtesy of Steris/Isomedix, Whippany, NJ.

flowing through the irradiator. It is then necessary to identify other products that have compatible densities and processing times. This is particularly cost effective if the manufacturer has product families of similar densities which can be run together at a single timer setting.

CRITICAL PROCESS PARAMETERS

The parameters used to determine acceptable dose delivery of gamma sterilization are as follows:

- cycle time
- product density
- loading pattern
- density mix

The parameters used to determine acceptable dose delivery of electron beam sterilization are as follows:

- beam energy
- beam current
- conveyor speed
- scan width
- product geometry
- product density

DOSE DISTRIBUTION

Dose rate is majorly different between E-beam and gamma sterilization because the mechanisms of interaction of gamma rays and electrons are different. Gamma ray penetration from two-sided dosing is relatively even with the min/max ratio close to one. Therefore, the process is not sensitive to small local changes in product thickness and density. In contrast, small changes in product thickness or density will cause the midline E-beam dose to rise or fall and will result in changes in the minimum to maximum (min/max) dose ratio. If the thickness is not uniform, the dose at the center will fall below the surface dose, and the min/max ratio will rise (Figure 6).

Dose delivery is also different, depending on many variables including the following:

- strength of the source
- penetration width
- size of the radiation field

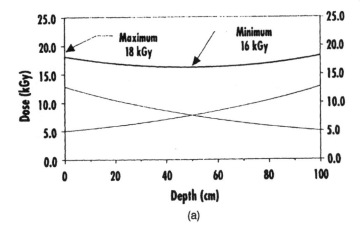

(a)

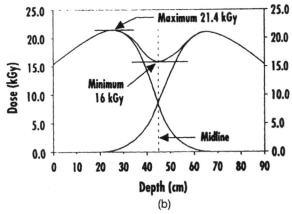

(b)

Figure 5 (a) Two-sided depth dose of cobalt 60 gamma rays in 1 m of a product with a 0.1 g/cm³ homogeneous density. A fraction of the energy passes through the product. (b) Two-sided depth dose of 10-MeV electrons in a 90-cm-thick product with a 0.1 g/cm³ homogeneous density. All the electron energy is absorbed in the product.

- distance of the product from the source
- product density
- type of radiation

For gamma, the dose rate near the source is in the range of 1–10 kGy/hour. Using sources with the same strength, the dose rate of an E-beam process will be many times greater than that of a gamma process, i.e., the average dose rate of a scanned beam is between 2–50 kGy/second. This faster absorption is achieved because the electron beam is unidirectional and is concentrated in a much smaller region and because the interaction of electrons with other electrons is much stronger than that of photons. The minimum radiation dose (D_{min}) and maximum radiation dose (D_{max}) will be determined largely by the total package configuration and the limitations of the irradiator. The target maximum dose (D_{max}) should produce a minimum amount of product degradation. The desired goal is to obtain a D_{max}/D_{min} ratio as close to 1 as possible.

DOSIMETERS

A dosimeter is a device that when irradiated exhibits a quantifiable change in some property of the device which can be related to the absorbed dose in a given material using appropriate analytical instrumentation and techniques (ASTM E170-97). Dosimeters are divided into various classes based on their relative quality and areas of application. Three types are used as standards—primary, reference, and transfer. The primary standard dosimeters are of the highest quality and are established and maintained by national standards laboratories. The two most commonly used are ionization chambers (International Commission of Radiation Units and Measurements) and calorimeters. Reference and transfer standard dosimeters are used to calibrate radiation sources and routine dosimeters (see Table 2, adapted from ISO 11137) used for routine measurement of absorbed dose. The reference dosimeter most widely used is the ferrous sulfate (Fricke) and dichromate aqueous solutions for gamma and the calorimeter for electron beam.

TABLE 2. Examples of Routine Dosimeters.

Dosimeter	Readout System	Approximate Absorbed Dose Range, kGy
Dyed polymethylmethacrylate	Visible spectrophotometer	10^3 to 5×10^4
Clear polymethylmethacrylate	Ultraviolet spectrophotometer	10^3 to 10^5
Cellulose triacetate	Ultraviolet spectrophotometer	10^4 to 4×10^5
Ceric-cerous sulfate solution	Potentiometer or ultraviolet spectrophotometer	10^3 to 10^5
Radiochromic dye film, solution, optical waveguide	Visible spectrophotometer or optical densiometer	1 to 10^5
Calorimeter*	Thermometer	10 to 10^5
Ferrous-cupric solution	Ultraviolet spectrophotometer	10^3 to 3×10^4

*Also a reference standard dosimeter.

Dosimetry systems consist of the dosimeter(s), measurement instruments, and their associated reference standards and procedures for the system's use. Selection of a suitable dosimeter system should take into consideration the following:

(1) Suitability of the dosimeter for the absorbed dose range of interest

(2) Adequate stability and reproducibility

(3) Ease of system calibration

(4) System calibration traceable to and consistent with national standards

(5) Ability to control or correct system response for systematic errors, such as those related to temperature and humidity

(6) Ease and simplicity of use

(7) Time and labor required for readout and interpretation

(8) Ruggedness of the system

(9) Variation of dosimeter response within a batch or between batches

(10) Effect of differences in radiation energy spectra between calibration and product irradiation fields

Each batch of dosimeters is calibrated by the irradiation of representative samples of dosimeters to known absorbed doses of radiation. This is accomplished by irradiation of the dosimeters at a standard or reference laboratory. Calibration procedures usually require the development of a calibration curve relating dosimeter response values to the absorbed dose. In practice, the curve is reduced to an equation from which tabulated values can be derived.

The following dosimeter characteristics may affect the uncertainty of the absorbed dose:

(1) Sensitivity to temperature

(2) Sensitivity to humidity—protect dosimeter from adverse conditions

(3) Dose rate dependence—a correction factor is applied if dosimeter is affected by rate

(4) Instability—absorbance may change over time

(5) Geometry—in the case of electron beam, geometry can introduce uncertainties

(6) Energy spectrum

(7) Reproducibility—dosimeters normally show random variability, so multiple dosimeters are used, and the variability is estimated by calculating standard deviation and the coefficient of variance.

DOSE MAPPING

Dose mapping of products in an established loading pattern is conducted to determine the minimum and maximum dose zones, the dose uniformity, and the processing rate (see Figure 7). The dose is determined using a dosimeter as described above. In general, when performing the dose map, the amount of product used should be the amount expected during typical irradiation runs. It is preferable to place dosimeters during dose mapping studies as follows:

- in regions of suspected high dose
- at interfaces between materials of different density
- at expected points of maximum buildup
- at points of suspected shadowing
- at points in all four quadrants
- at the dose monitoring point to be used during routine processing

The key objectives of the dose map are to locate the maximum and minimum internal doses within the product (load) and relate them to the dose at the reference point. Once determined, the internal max/min can be predicted simply by measuring the reference point.

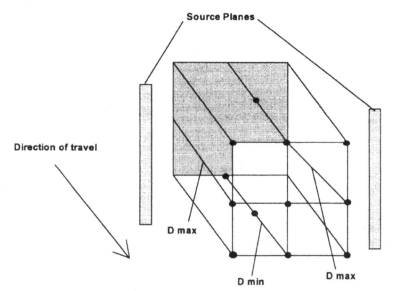

Figure 7 Dose mapping—gamma.

The contractor or in-house sterilization manager is responsible for performing these studies and for maintaining the calibration of the dosimeters. During routine processing, the manufacturer must maintain the load configuration density as mapped in order to ensure proper dosing. If the load (case density) density changes, a new dose map should be determined. Also, if the gamma facility adds additional isotope to the irradiator or changes the distribution of the isotope in the source rack, the processing rate changes, and a new dose map should be performed to confirm the new operating characteristics.

The manufacturer can monitor the radiation processing characteristics over time by charting the measured maximum (D_{max}) and minimum (D_{min}) dose for a defined product group over time. Variations in the dose should be small over time, indicating that the device load and bulk density are well-defined and maintained, that the irradiator operators have been precise in the placement of the dosimeters, and that members of the facility's staff have reproduced the appropriate dwell times and followed the correct procedures.

CHAPTER 3

Contract Sterilization

THE medical device industry is using contract sterilization at an increasing rate. A contractual relationship must exist between the manufacturer and the sterilization contractor in order to guarantee a well-controlled sterilization process capable of producing a sterile, safe, and effective product. A direct impact of this trend is a downsizing of the sterilization support and technical knowledge within the medical device manufacturer's staff. Proper communication and understanding of the sterilizer's activities is essential. The responsibility for sterility is therefore shared, and the division of responsibilities must be clearly defined and understood by both parties. A partial list of contract sterilization facilities is included in Appendix 1.

Validation of the sterilizing dose is the responsibility of the device manufacturer, but responsibility for the validation tasks may be delegated to individuals employed by the contractor. Even if the contractor assumes responsibility for the validation, the device manufacturer is still ultimately responsible for the safety and efficacy of those devices it produces. Contract sterilizers are considered an extension of the device manufacturer's operation and are responsible for the manufacturing operations that they perform.

Even before the sterilization facility is chosen, a decision must be made as to what will be the most appropriate sterilization method. Even though some sterilization contractors perform both ethylene oxide and radiation sterilization, the choice of the most appropriate method for your product and package is still the first important step. Table 3 contains some significant considerations, but certainly not all that will help with this decision.

19

TABLE 3. Considerations for Selection of Appropriate Sterilization Method.

Consideration	Ethylene Oxide	Radiation
Device materials	Compatible with most materials; maximum temperature tolerance of 120–130°F; can use 100–120°F, but less effective	Selection of suitable grades of plastics to prevent degradation over time after exposure to maximum dose ranges
Device design	Must allow penetration of gas and humidity into interior spaces	No restrictions
Device package	Must be permeable to gas and humidity and allow aeration after cycle completion	No restrictions
Post sterile time	3–7 day quarantine for BI release and EtO gas dissipation	Dosimetric release

SELECTION OF THE STERILIZATION FACILITY

To adequately determine the contractor's acceptability and to satisfy the QSR requirement 21 CFR Sec. 820.50(a), the manufacturer should perform an audit using a person who is knowledgeable about the sterilization method being considered. The audit should be performed following a predetermined audit procedure. Once completed, the auditor should prepare a written report stating the contractor's acceptability and any corrective actions deemed necessary. The audit should cover the following:

- maintenance and calibration
- installation qualification
- equipment documentation including irradiator specifications and characteristics, location of the radiator with respect to segregation of nonirradiated from irradiated products, description and operation of conveyor systems, dimensions of irradiation containers, description of the manner of operation of the irradiator, and location and certification of source materials in a gamma facility
- personnel training
- change control and documentation procedures
- quality systems
- software validation
- dosimeter calibration
- compliance with local regulators and safety procedures

OBTAIN A WRITTEN CONTRACT

Requirements for a written contract when interstate shipping is involved are found in 21 Code of Federal Regulations 801.150(e); for intrastate services, a contract is recommended to ensure compliance with QSR 21 CFR 820.181. The written agreement should outline the services and procedures to be supplied and followed by both parties. For radiation sterilization, the written agreement should contain at least the following:

(1) Information transfer—specify individuals responsible for coordinating the flow of information

(2) Records—specify required documentation to be used and maintained

(3) Process validation—specify all parameters with tolerances to be qualified and the criteria for requalification

(4) Loading configuration—specify minimum and maximum number of totes, tote loading, packaging, load wrapping for shipment, minimum sterilization dose, location of test samples (if used), and dosimeters

(5) Types of dosimeters used and maintenance, calibration, and storage procedures

(6) Minimum dose specification and process control—specify dose that should be achieved once validation is complete and specify acceptable tolerances

(7) Post-sterilization handling—specify procedures for release of product and for shipment

(8) Batch record and review—specify procedure and responsibility for approving sterilization batch records prior to release

(9) Finished product release—specify procedures and identify individuals responsible for approving release

(10) Audits—specify scope of audits, corrective actions, documentation of audit, and confidentiality

(11) Change control, process deviations, and product damage—specify individuals to be notified of any changes or deviations or product damage

(12) Reprocessing of loads—specify how reprocessing procedures are established, implemented, and controlled to assure that the steps meet the validation and routine processing specifications

(13) Material handling and documentation—specify how adherence to label control is conducted

(14) Contract agreement criteria—specify all shipping requirements including labeling for shipping and identify laboratories to be used for sample testing

VERIFICATION OF VALIDATION

The validation documentation from the contract sterilizer is the same as the documentation required if performing the studies in-house and should include the following:

(1) Sterilization process information
- minimum dose delivered
- dose map
- dose min/max ratio
- timer setting

(2) Documents
- validation protocol approved by manufacturer and contract sterilizer
- final report approved by manufacturer and contract sterilizer
- written agreement between manufacturer and contractor

(3) Product information
- list of products or product families included in the validation
- tote loading to include sample placement
- lots and quantity of products used
- description of product and test samples, if any
- rationale for development of product families
- rationale for selection of process challenge device and SIP (if used)

(4) Dosimeter placement
- locations within the product load
- dose map for every load configuration or every different product density

(5) Equipment testing (calibration) and documentation
- gamma—critical process parameters including timer setting, exposure time or conveyor speed, and dose measurements
- E-beam—electron beam characteristics such as current, energy, scan width, conveyor speed, and dose measurements

- dose mapping of irradiator to characterize magnitude, distribution, and reproducibility of dose delivery

(6) Other information
- bioburden information
- product and packaging functionality test results
- product sterility test results
- statement of acceptance
- material compatibility and biocompatibility (if new material)
- pyrogen test results (if blood contacting)
- bacteriostasis/fungistasis test results

ROUTINE PROCESSING

Once the validation is completed successfully, routine processing can begin. The manufacturer is responsible for properly preparing the load and the accompanying instructions as follows:

- The product is packaged to maintain product integrity and cleanliness.
- The quantity of product and test samples is documented.
- Each pallet, carton, or designated shipper is marked to show its nonsterile nature, e.g., "Nonsterile: Shipped for further processing."
- Products shipped have a validated process and minimum dose specification.
- The contract sterilizer is provided with instructions for handling products that are damaged.
- The number of pallets, lot number of products, and quality of product per lot are identified on each pallet, and the total number is documented in the shipping papers.
- Include instructions for sample placement, retrieval, and shipping to the designated test lab, if required.
- Include directions on post-sterilization handling and shipping times.

Once the contractor receives the load, it is processed according to the validated process specifications. In addition, the contractor is responsible for the following:

(1) Documenting the quantity of product and test samples received
(2) Processing and reporting any deviations from specification

(3) Segregating product to avoid mixing sterile and nonsterile product
(4) Documenting material damage
(5) Reviewing records to ensure compliance with specification
(6) Recording the effect of process interruptions
(7) Dose monitoring—placement and retrieval
(8) Shipping product loads with identifying labels on each pallet containing the designation: "Sterilized—Awaiting test results"
(9) Providing the following documentation:
   - test sample (if used) and dosimeter placement and retrieval information
   - lot number, quality received, sterilized, and shipped
   - sterilization batch number and date
   - specified dose received and maximum dose
   - written release or acceptance of the sterilization processing records
   - documentation of any damage, deviations, and changes that could affect the process

On receipt of the routine batch information from the contractor, the manufacturer should review the processing documentation to ensure that the validated specifications were met. The device history file for each product lot is prepared by including with the approved processing records the sterility test results (if a dose audit), other test results (if stipulated), any product or package inspection results, and reconciliation of product lot quantities. If all records are in order, the sterilization load is released to finished goods. A qualified person reviews any deviations that may have occurred and the appropriate investigation or corrective action performed and documented.

CHAPTER 4

Prevalidation Planning

PRODUCT AND PACKAGE MATERIALS EVALUATION

PRIOR to the application of radiation for sterilization of a product, the effect of the radiation on the materials that make up the products and packaging must be considered. Guidance on selecting a test is available in AAMI TIR 17: 1997, *Radiation sterilization—Material qualification*. The loss of functional properties is often the most important result of polymer irradiation. Properties affected can include the following:

- tensile strength
- impact strength
- shear strength
- elongation

For pharmaceutical products, response of a drug must be understood. No unique radiolytic products have been found in irradiated drugs. The breakdown products found after irradiation are identical to those found during manufacture of a drug, or are metabolites of the drug. Newer techniques for irradiating drugs require that drugs be treated in a frozen state because water, which comprises the bulk of a parenteral or oral drug, is the major source of free radicals resulting from bombardment with gamma photons or electrons. Freezing takes advantage of the fact that any free radicals formed become trapped in the ice crystal structure, thereby producing less damage.

All materials break down at high radiation doses; below the destructive levels, however, the dose necessary to produce significant property changes can differ depending on the polymer material and its

25

chemical structure. This depends on whether polymer scission (causing reduced toughness and elongation) or cross-linking (causing increased strength and stiffness) occurs. The majority of polymers used are radiation stable at doses typically used to sterilize health care products. However, all polymer selections should be thoroughly challenged in the specific application and processing conditions. Ta-

TABLE 4. Relative Radiation Stability of Medical Polymer "Families."

Dose (Kilogray) in Ambient Air at which Elongation Decreases by 25%

NOTE: This chart represents the best available data as of this date and is intended as a guidance, specific resin formulations must be evaluated in the intended application for the effects of radiation and; (1) residual & functional stress, (2) section thickness (3) molecular weight & distribution, (4) morphology (5) environment (oxygen/temperature) (6) dose rate

Legend*
1 - HDPE
2 - PBT
3 - Aromatic
4 - Rigid/Semi - Rigid PVC
5 - ETFE (Tefzel)
6 - Hi-Impacy ABS
7 - Butyl Rubber
8 - Silicone/Neoprene
9 - EPDM
10 - Nylon 8 & 12
11 - Amorphous Nylon
12 - Cellulose/Paper
13 - PMMA
14 - Varies by MfgrGrade
15 - Homopolymer

REFERENCES:
* Polymer Manufacturers Data
* NASA/Jet Propulsion Laboratories, "Effects of Radiation on Polymers & Elastomers", 1988
* Skeins & Williams,"Ionizing Radiation Effect on Selected Biomedical Polymers"
* Kiang, "Effect of Gamma Irradiation on Elastomeric Closures, PDA, 1992
* Ley, "The Effects of Irradiation on Packaging Materials", 1976

*Within each family is a range of radiation stabilities, the "steps" are intended to show significant family members.
Courtesy of Karl J. Hemmerich, Ageless Processing Technologies.

TABLE 5. Relative Radiation Stability of Medical Polymers.

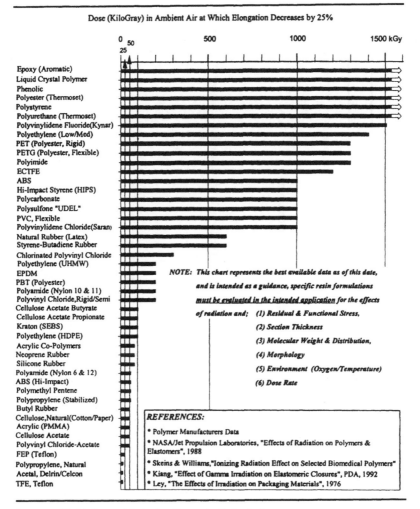

Dose (KiloGray) in Ambient Air at Which Elongation Decreases by 25%

NOTE: *This chart represents the best available data as of this date, and is intended as a guidance, specific resin formulations* must be evaluated in the intended application *for the effects of radiation and; (1) Residual & Functional Stress,*

(2) Section Thickness

(3) Molecular Weight & Distribution,

(4) Morphology

(5) Environment (Oxygen/Temperature)

(6) Dose Rate

REFERENCES:

* Polymer Manufacturers Data
* NASA/Jet Propulsion Laboratories, "Effects of Radiation on Polymers & Elastomers", 1988
* Skeins & Williams,"Ionizing Radiation Effect on Selected Biomedical Polymers"
* Kiang, "Effect of Gamma Irradiation on Elastomeric Closures", PDA, 1992
* Ley, "The Effects of Irradiation on Packaging Materials", 1976

Courtesy of Karl J. Hemmerich, Ageless Processing Technologies.

bles 4 and 5 summarize information available from government, industry, and scientific studies concerning radiation effects on polymer properties after exposure to various doses. These tables graphically display the dose at which a number of common plastics experience a 25% loss in elongation. Loss of elongation is a commonly used measure of the effect of radiation. A more qualitative summary is given in Table 6.

TABLE 6. General Guide to Radiation Stability of Materials.

Materials	Radiation Stability	Comments
Thermoplastics		
ABS	Good	High impact grades are not as radiation resistant as standard impact grades.
Acrylics (PMMA)	Fair/good	
Cellulosics		
Esters	Fair	Esters degrade less than cellulose.
Cellulose acetate propionate	Fair	
Cellulose acetate butyrate	Good/fair	
Cellulose, paper, cardboard	Fair/good	
Fluoropolymers		
Polytetrafluoroethylene (PTFE)	Poor	When irradiated, PTFE and PFA are significantly damaged. The others show better stability.
Perfluoro alkoxy (PFA)	Poor	
Polychlorotrifluoroethylene (PCTFE)	Good/excellent	
Polyvinyl fluoride (PVF)	Good/excellent	
Polyvinylidene fluoride (PVDF)	Good/excellent	
Ethylene-tetrafluoroethylene (ETFE)	Good	
Fluorinated ethylene propylene (FEP)	Fair	
Liquid crystal polymer (LCP)	Excellent	Commercial LCPs; natural LCPs are not stable.
Polyacetals	Poor	Irradation causes embrittlement. Color changes have been noted (yellow to green).
Polyamides (nylon)	Good	Nylon 10, 11, 12, 6-6, more stable than 6. Nylon film and fibers are less resistant.
Polycarbonate	Good/excellent	Yellows—mechanical properties not greatly affected; color-correction formulas are available.
Polyesters	Good/excellent	PBT not as stable at PET resins.
Polyethylene, various densities	Good/excellent	HD not as stable as MD and LD.

28

TABLE 6. (continued).

Materials	Radiation Stability	Comments
Polyimides	Excellent	
Polyphenylene sulfide	Excellent	
Polypropylene, natural	Poor-fair	Physical properties are greatly reduced when irradiated. Radiation stabilizes grades utilizing high M_w and copolymerized and alloyed with polyethylene, should be used
Polypropylene, stabilized		in most applications. High-dose-rate E-beam may reduce oxidative degradation.
Polystyrene	Excellent	
Polysulfone	Excellent	Natural material is yellow.
Polyurethane	Excellent/good	Aromatic discolors; polyesters more stable than esters. Retains physical properties.
Polyvinylchloride (PVC)	Good	Yellows—antioxidants and stabilizers prevent yellowing. High M_w organotin stabilizers improve stability; color-correctd radiation formulas available.
Polyvinylchloride-Polyvinylacetate	Good	Less resistant than PVC.
Polyvinylidene-dichloride (Saran)	Good	Less resistant than PVC.
Styrene/Acrylonitrile (SAN)	Good/excellent	
Elastomers		
Butyl	Poor	Friable; sheds particles.
Chlorosulfonated polyethylene	Poor	
EDPM	Excellent	
Natural rubber	Good/excellent	Discolors.
Nitrile	Good/excellent	
Polyacrylic	Poor	
Polychloroprene (neoprene)	Good	Discolors; addition of aromatic plasticizers renders material more stable.

(continued)

29

TABLE 6. (continued).

Materials	Radiation Stability	Comments
Silicone	Good	Phenyl-methyl silicones are more stable than methyl silicones. Full cure during manufacture can eliminate most post-radiation effects.
Styrene-butadiene	Good	
Urethane	Excellent	
Thermosets		
Allyl diglycol carbonate	Excellent	Maintains excellent optical properties.
Epoxies	Excellent	All curing systems.
Phenolics	Excellent	Includes the addition of mineral fillers.
Polyesters	Excellent	Includes the addition of mineral and glass fibers.
Polyurethanes		
Aliphatic	Excellent	
Aromatic	Good/excellent	Darkening can occur. Possible breakdown products could be derived

Adapted from International Atomic Energy Agency, 1990.

ACCELERATED AGING

The effects of radiation on packaging and product materials (see Table 7) might not be immediately apparent. Accelerated aging studies expose sterile devices (and/or the packaging) to exaggerated stress or stresses in order to predict the effects of normal stress or stresses on the future functionality and reliability of a product or package (see Appendix 9 for a generic protocol). Using this method results in lower product development costs and earlier product introduction that benefits the patient and the company. Since this is only a predictor of performance, ambient aging should also be performed for a period of time typical of the product's shelf life. Products should be exposed to doses higher than expected for routine sterilization, and nonirradiated controls should be included in the program. A typical program could include devices or material samples exposed at various dose levels between 20–30 and 100 kGy.

A single stressor is typically used: temperature. Aging studies work best when moderate aging temperatures (<60°C) are selected, i.e., temperatures below the point at which product distortion is produced (10°C less than any major thermal transitions). One of the most widely used techniques for estimating future properties of medical materials (method outlined in AAMI TIR 17, *Radiation sterilization—Material qualification*) is based on the work of Arrhenius who established a relationship between temperature and reaction rate: the aging rate (Q) will double for every 10°C that the temperature is raised. The Q_{10} method assumes that the ratio of the time to equivalent damage at low temperature (usually 10°C apart) has a constant value. The Q_{10} value will decrease with increasing temperatures. This approximation ($Q_{10} = 2$) is used in the simplest protocols for estimating a conservative aging factor (AF).

$$AF = Q_{10}^{(T_{T1} - T_{RT})/10}$$

where

Q_{10} = rate of chemical reaction
T_{T1} = high temperature (test temperature)
T_{RT} = low temperature (ambient)

The AF can then be used to determine the appropriate accelera-

TABLE 7. Typical Mechanisms of Degradation.

- loss of volatile constituents
- oxidation enhancing chain session
- continuing molecular polymerization
- hydrolytic cleavage by reaction with moisture
- chemical breakdown of constituents and formation of degradation products
- consumption of heat stabilizers or antioxidants

tion aging time based on the expected or predicted shelf life as follows:

$$T_{T1} = T_{RT} / AF$$

where

T_{T1} = oven aging temperature
T_{RT} = normal environmental temperature

Example: Accelerated aging time needed for five years shelf life claim:

$$T_{T1} = 60°C$$

$$T_{RT} = 22°C$$

$$Q_{10} = 2$$

$$T_{T1} = \frac{260 \text{ wks}}{2^{(60-22)/10}} = \frac{260}{2^{3.8}} = \frac{260}{13.94} = 18.7 \text{ weeks}$$

Figure 8 shows the relationship between the aging temperature and equivalency to a one-year room temperature aging using various Q_{10} values.

There are no published standards for performing an accelerated aging study. The *USP* has a section <1191> entitled "Stability Considerations in Dispensing Practice" that supplies general information. It includes a list of five sets of criteria for acceptable levels of stability for drug products as follows:

(1) Chemical
(2) Physical
(3) Microbiological

(4) Therapeutic
(5) Toxicological

   The American Society for Testing and Materials (ASTM) standard, "Standard Guide for Accelerated Aging of Sterile Medical Device Packages" provides information for developing accelerated aging protocols to rapidly determine the effects due to the passage of time and environmental effects on the sterile integrity of packages and condones the simplified Q_{10} method.
   Basic protocol steps would include the following (see Appendix 9):

• Understand product environment, materials, and primary constituents of deteriorative reactions.

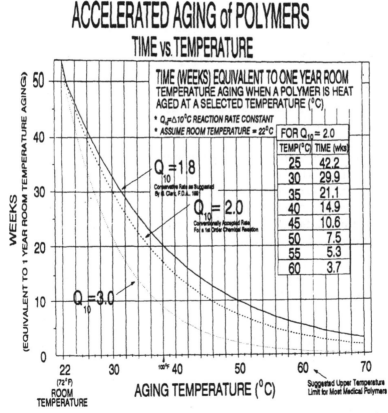

Figure 8 Relationship of time vs. temperature for accelerated aging studies (adapted from Hemmerich, 1998).

- Establish reaction rates and order of reaction.
- Assume applicability of Arrhenius relationship.
- Establish maximum aging temperature based on keeping the polymer in the same physical state as the service environment and not altering reactants.
- Establish time for volatilization of absorbed gases, liquids, plasticizers, additives, etc.
- Record kinetic data while being aware of problems with initial data and low conversions.
- Correlate data to initial expression and adjust to changes in concentrations and order.
- Determine the Arrhenius parameters and their accuracy.
- Extrapolate rate parameters to service conditions and integrate to predict behavior with time.

Basic radiation application guidelines that may apply are as follows:

- Most polymers are durable at the radiation doses typically used for sterilization. All materials should be carefully evaluated over the product's shelf life.
- All polymers, both scission and cross-link—those that cross-link more than scission generally do better in the radiation environment.
- Aromatic materials are more radiation resistant than aliphatic materials. The benzene ring structure present in an aromatic compound acts as a stabilizer, rearranging itself to accept or donate an electron as needed.
- Antioxidants and UV stabilizers improve radiation resistance; the impact of these additives on biocompatibility should be considered.
- The highest molecular weight material possible for the application (with the most narrow molecular weight distribution) should be used.
- Amorphous materials provide better radiation enhancement when compared to semicrystalline materials. For semicrystalline materials, higher amorphous content provides better radiation enhancement.
- Materials with low oxygen permeability are more radiation resistant.
- Materials used in thin films and fibers should be selected with

caution due to the enhanced effect of oxidation resulting from the large surface-to-mass ratio.

• Effects of radiation on polymers are generally cumulative with each subsequent exposure of the product.

There are many tests used in materials evaluation; a selection of those is shown in Table 8. Once a material is selected on the basis of these tests, final qualification to demonstrate full functionality should be carried out on fully processed components and complete devices and packages.

TABLE 8. Physical and Functional Test Methods for Plastic Material Evaluation.

Test	Test Method	Test Reference
Embrittlement		
Tensile properties	Tensile strength	ISO/R 527: 1996
	Ultimate elongation	ISO/R 527: 1996
	Modulus of elasticity	ISO/R 527: 1996
	Work	ISO/R 527: 1996
Flexural properties	Flange bending test	"Stability of Irradiated Polypropylene. 1. Mechanical Properties," Williams, Dunn, Sugg, Stannet, *Advances in Chemistry* Series, No. 169, Stabilization and Degradation of Polymers, Eds. Allara, Hawkins, pp. 142–150, 1978.
	Flexbar test	ISO 178: 1975
	Impact resistance	1985 ASTM Standards, Vol. 08.01—Plastics, D-785-65
Hardness	Shore	ISO 868: 1985
	Rockwell	1985 ASTM Standards, Vol. 08.01—Plastics, D-785-65
	Compression strength	ISO 604: 1973
	Burst strength	1985 ASTM Standards, Vol. 08.01—Plastics (Tubing), D-1180-57
	Tear strength	1985 ASTM Standards, Vol. 08.01—Plastics, D-1004-66, and ISO 6383/1, 1983
Tests for discoloration	Yellowness index	1985 ASTM Standards, Vol. 08.01—Plastics, D-1925-70
	Optical spectrometry	1985 ASTM Standards, Vol. 08.01—Plastics, D-1746-70

Adapted from International Atomic Energy Agency, 1990.

ESTABLISHMENT AND MAINTENANCE OF PRODUCT FAMILIES

For efficient and cost-effective validation performance, prior product and process evaluation is suggested. If your company produces a wide range of sterile products, similar devices can be grouped into families. A family of products can be considered to be all those products of similar design and materials of construction, but consisting of different sizes, i.e., all Foley catheters, sized 8 French to 16 French, and similar bioburden levels. After family groups are determined, select the most difficult-to-sterilize representative product in the family to represent all of the devices in the group. Generally, this device will have the highest and most resistant bioburden population. If your evaluation results in multiple product families, it is advisable to select from the representative products, a single most-difficult-to-sterilize product that will be used as the master process challenge device (PCD). Guidance for evaluation of products can be found in AAMI TIR 15843: 1998, *Sterilization of health care products—Radiation sterilization—Product families, sampling plans for verification dose experiments and sterilization dose audits, and frequency of sterilization dose audits.*

GROUPING INTO PRODUCT FAMILIES

Product families for radiation processing are based on bioburden. Bioburden histories for individual products should be maintained over time. In addition, assessment of individual products and their similarities should be considered as well as the impact of the variables shown below on the bioburden. Document your review and the rationale for placement of devices into families and create a final family listing including the device name and catalog (part) number. This can become part of the protocol or be incorporated into a standard operating procedure (SOP).

After evaluation of bioburden populations, examples of product-related variables to consider include the following:

- raw materials
- components
- product design and size
- manufacturing process
- manufacturing equipment

- manufacturing environment
- manufacturing location

SELECTION OF FAMILY REPRESENTATIVE

Each family of products will contain a number of devices. From these devices, the representative challenge product is selected. The selected device will be the most difficult device to sterilize in the family group and will be used in verification dose experiments. A simulated product not intended for sale can be used as long as it is made of similar materials and uses similar manufacturing processes as the actual product. The establishment and continued validity of the sterilization dose are related to numbers and resistances of organisms on or in the product. This is the basic characteristic used to select the representative product. Other criteria that should be considered by a knowledgeable person when selecting the challenge product are as follows:

- number of microorganisms
- types of microorganisms
- size of product
- number of components
- complexity of product
- degree of automation during manufacture (manually assembled products will generally have higher bioburden levels)
- manufacturing environment

Modifications to products, such as raw materials, components, or product design, and changes to the manufacturing process, facility, or environment should be formally evaluated and documented to assess their effect on bioburden levels and dose validation. Bioburden data should be collected on an established time frame for all products within the family to ensure that the selected representative product continues to be the most difficult to sterilize item in the group.

SELECTION OF A SAMPLE ITEM PORTION (SIP)

Whenever possible, the entire product should be used for testing. Selection of items for dose setting is based on the individual product unit (Table 9). A product unit can include the following:

(1) An individual product within its primary package

TABLE 9. Selection of Items for Dose Setting.

Product Unit	Item for Bioburden Estimation or Incremental Dose Experiment	Item for Verification Experiment	Basis for Sterilization Dose	Rationale
Individual health care product in its primary package	Individual health care product	Individual health care product	Individual health care product	Each health care product is used independently in clinical practice
Set of components in primary package	Combination of components	Combination of components	Combination of components	Components are assembled as a product and used together in clinical practice
Number of identical products in primary package	Single health care product taken from primary package	Single health care product taken from primary package	Single health care product taken from primary package	Each health care product is used independently in clinical practice
Kit of procedure-related health care products	Each type of individual item tested separately	Each type of individual item tested separately	Highest sterilization dose of the individual items	Each health care product is used independently in clinical practice

Adapted from Amendment 1 to AAMI/ISO 11137 : 1994.

(2) A set of components presented in a primary package that is assembled at the point of use
(3) A number of identical products within a primary package
(4) A kit composed of a variety of procedure-related products

Testing an entire product is not always possible due to product size or complexity. In such situations, a sample portion of the product unit (SIP) that is easy to handle during testing may be selected. The SIP should be as large a portion of the product unit as is possible to manipulate readily in the laboratory. SIPs can be selected based on length, weight, and volume or surface area of the product, as appropriate.

The SIP should represent the microbial challenge of the entire product unit. That is, if the distribution of viable organisms on the product is uniform, then any portion of the product can be used. In the absence of this information, the SIP can be composed of several different portions of the product unit selected at random. Remember that after exposure to a verification dose, the SIP must be transferred into a sterility test medium. The fewer the number of manipulations or transfers required during this test, the lower the chance of inadvertent contamination. The SIP may be divided into two or more containers if too large to fit into one, but again, the number of transfers per product unit should be minimized. The SIP should be prepared and packaged to minimize alteration of the bioburden.

The appropriateness of the SIP selection should be determined by performing a sterility test using 20 SIPs following ISO 11737-2. At least seventeen of these tests should be positive. Examples of SIP selection excerpted from ISO 11737-2 are outlined in Table 10.

SIPs for kits containing multiples of the same product are based on a single product and not on the summation of all of the products in the kit. For example, if a kit contains five syringes and one syringe is

TABLE 10. Basis for Selection of a Sample Item Portion (SIP).

Basis for SIP Selection	Product Examples
Surface area	Implants (nonabsorbable)
Mass	Powders
	Surgical gowns/drapes
	Implants (absorbable)
Length	Tubing (consistent diameter)
Volume	Water, fluids
Fluid path	Intravenous delivery sets, fluid bags

tested, then the syringe SIP = 1. For kits containing a variety of products, the SIP is based upon each type of product, and a separate SIP is established for each product in the kit. For example, if a kit contains two gowns, two towels, two pairs of gloves, and a drape, then individual SIPs are determined for each product independent of the other products in the kit.

A SIP can also be used if the device under evaluation is very costly. The manufacturer may decide that instead of using 100 complete units, each device should be divided into five portions equal in anticipated bioburden levels, both in numbers and types. Twenty such devices would then yield 100 SIPs equal to 0.2% of the original device.

STERILITY ASSURANCE LEVELS (SAL)

The selection of an appropriate sterility assurance level (SAL) is dependent on the intended use of the product and the ability of the product to withstand a terminal sterilization process. The SAL is based on the bacterial survival curve (Figure 9). When a population of microbial cells is irradiated, the number of viable cells in the population diminishes exponentially as the radiation dose increases to a point where no viable cells remain. The D_{10} value for a particular organism is the dose required to reduce a population to 10% of its initial value. When applied to SAL, the terms "higher than" and "greater than" mean that there is a higher assurance of sterility, which provides a lower probability of a surviving organism in a population of product units (e.g., a 10^{-6} SAL is greater than a 10^{-3} SAL).

Together with knowledge of the original bioburden, the D_{10} value is used to calculate the dose required to achieve a given SAL. For terminally sterilized products to be labeled "sterile," the theoretical probability of a surviving organism present on the product can be either 10^{-3} or 10^{-6}, depending on the intended use of the product. For products intended for distribution in the U.S. only, a dual sterility assurance level is acceptable (documented in AAMI Draft ST 67, *Sterilization of medical devices—Requirements for products labeled "sterile"*), whereas for products for sale in the EU, the requirement for terminally sterilized products is a SAL of 10^{-6} (documented in EN 556: *Sterilization of medical devices—Requirements for medical devices to be labeled sterile*). The decision to select a SAL less than 10^{-6} can be considered when the product:

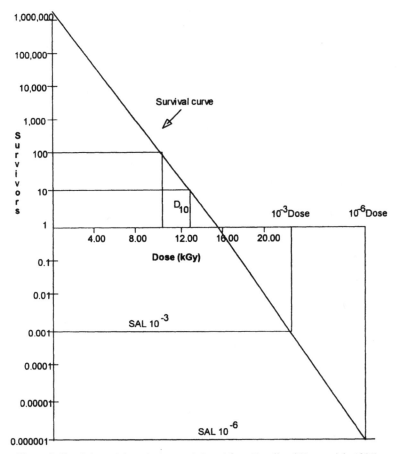

Figure 9 Simple bacterial survival curve (adapted from Farrell and Hemmerich, 1995).

(1) Cannot be designed to allow a sterilization process that achieves a SAL of 10^{-6} without adversely affecting its essential safety and function

(2) Offers unique benefits for patient diagnosis, treatment, or care

(3) Is unique insofar as there exists no alternative product for the same purpose that can be sterilized with a process that achieves a 10^{-6} SAL

When applicable, the product must be sterilized using a validated process where the theoretical probability of a microorganism surviving is a SAL of 10^{-5}, then 10^{-4} or 10^{-3}.

A 10^{-6} SAL would be appropriate for the following:

(1) Products intended to come into contact with compromised tissue
   - wound dressing
   - cardiac catheters
   - cauterizing devices
   - scalpels and other surgical instruments
   - surgeon's gloves
   - syringes
   - hypodermic needles
   - parenteral solutions
   - peritoneal dialysis solutions
   - prefilled syringes
   - laparotomy sponges
   - incise drapes

(2) Products with claims of sterile fluid pathway
   - fluid pathways of IV sets
   - fluid pathways of syringes
   - collection containers or bags

(3) Surgically implanted devices
   - reconstructive devices (e.g., hip, elbow, knee)
   - active implantable devices
   - trauma devices (e.g., nails, screws, plates, pins, wires, etc.)
   - sutures
   - intraocular lenses

A 10^{-3} SAL is appropriate for products not intended to come into contact with compromised tissue, such as the following:

(1) Specimen collection or transfer devices
   - blood collection tubes for *in vitro* diagnostic tests
   - culture media devices
   - serological pipettes
   - specimen containers

(2) Topical devices
   - ECG electrodes
   - drainage bags
   - grounding pads
   - surgical drapes and gowns

(3) Mucosal contacting devices
- tongue depressors
- examination gloves
- urinary catheters

(4) Non-fluid path surfaces of sterile devices
- external surface of IV sets

(5) Products that cannot withstand a 10^{-6} SAL process
- porcine heart valve
- wound dressings of a biological nature

CHAPTER 5

Microbiological Considerations

$\mathbf{M}$ ICROBIOLOGISTS are familiar with the concept that bacteria subjected to a sterilizing agent will, in theory, die exponentially with time at a uniform rate. A constant percentage of the microbial population is inactivated with each successive time interval. The absorbed dose required to destroy 90%, or one (1) log, of the microbial population is defined as the D_{10} value, or decimal reduction value. Therefore, a semi-log plot (Figure 9) will yield a straight-line relationship. Note that when the line crosses below 10^0, resulting in less than one survivor, it is expressed as a probability of survival. Thus, the 10^{-6} survivor level or sterility assurance level (SAL) or a 12-spore log reduction (SLR) represents a one-in-one million probability of one microorganism surviving the process.

EVALUATION OF PRODUCT BIOBURDEN

Bioburden is the population of viable microorganisms on a raw material, a component of a finished device. It is the result of the materials and components from which the product was made and how it was manufactured. Factors that can influence bioburden are as follows:

- raw materials—synthetic (lower) vs. natural origin (higher)
- manufacturing of components—molding or casting (lower) vs. hand cutting (higher)
- level of control in the manufacturing environment
- assembly/manufacturing aids—compressed air, water, lubricants
- cleaning prior to packaging (reduces numbers)
- packaging of finished products—manual (higher) vs. automated (lower)

45

An understanding of the viable microorganisms on a finished device is necessary and required to support the validation process. Bioburden data are important because the extent of the treatment of a sterilization process is a function of the bioburden on the product, the resistance of the bioburden, and the sterility assurance level required. The assessment of the bioburden needs to include the number of microorganisms with their identities. The identification need not be exhaustive, but confirmation of Gram stain characteristics and genus provide useful information and can be used to monitor changes over time and as a comparison to organisms recovered during environmental monitoring. Bioburden ranges typically found on device types are illustrated in Table 11.

If your company has a large number of products, it may be difficult and time consuming to test each one. Again, grouping into families will address the requirement of knowing the bioburden levels by allowing actual testing of only the selected family representative. To obtain the appropriate family representative, consider the material of construction (natural materials usually contain the higher numbers of microorganisms), the device size (choose the largest in a group of similar products), or a complicated device (one containing a number of assembled subcomponents). The adhesion of microorganisms to different materials will vary considerably. Some examples of different bioburden levels encountered on different types of products are illustrated in Figure 10.

Perform the bioburden evaluation by selecting ten packaged devices randomly from one (1) lot of recently manufactured product. If devices are costly, decrease the number sampled to five (5). A simulated product can be used but must be made from the same materials and in the same manufacturing process. Products rejected during the manufacturing process can also be used as long as they were exposed

TABLE 11. Bioburden Load Ranges.

Relative Bioburden	Generic Products	Specifics
Low	Metal devices	Laparoscopic cannulas, needles
	Extruded plastics and synthetics	Catheters, syringes, tubing
	Plastics, synthetics	Sutures
	Bleached fabrics, partially automated	Dressings
	Natural materials/treated	Cotton stockinet
High	Natural materials/untreated	Heterographs

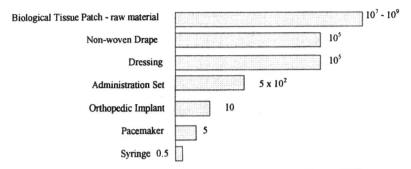

Figure 10 Magnitude of bioburden on devices (adapted from Hoxey, 1993).

to all process steps. Do not use expired or "old" product for bioburden evaluation, because the organisms on such products may not represent those present on recently manufactured products. The frequency of the bioburden estimations, supported by documented evidence or rationale, should be established based on several factors including the following:

- data from previous bioburden estimates [if historical data is consistent, less frequent testing is indicated (for example, shift from monthly to quarterly or semi-annually)]
- use to be made of the bioburden data
- manufacturing processes
- batch size
- production frequency for the product
- materials used (change in materials may trigger new bioburden estimate)
- variations in the bioburden estimates (spikes or swings in data could signal more frequent testing)

The test method used only produces an estimate of the number of microorganisms. The method should be validated to establish the relationship between the estimate and the true number of microorganisms on the product. Whatever method is used must be reproducible so that the results generated on one occasion can be compared to data generated subsequently. The method of extraction most effective for bioburden recovery varies according to the substrate; therefore, individual products may require different extraction methods to optimize organism removal. All treatments should avoid conditions that are likely to affect the viability of the microorganism, such as excessive cavitation, shear forces, temperature rises, or osmotic shock. Guidance on acceptable bioburden recovery methods is available in ANSI/AAMI/ISO 11737-1: 1995, *Sterilization of medical devices—microbiological methods—Part 1: Estimation of population of microorganisms on product.*

The estimation of the bioburden can be divided into three phases, all of which may affect the final results and therefore should be considered in the validation:

(1) The removal of the microorganism from the device—extraction techniques could include use of ultrasonication, mechanical agitation with or without glass beads, vortex mixing, flushing, blending, swabbing, and contact plating and stomaching. A surfactant may be used in the extraction fluid to facilitate removal of organisms.

(2) Transfer of the organisms to the cultural conditions quickly— methods could include membrane filtration, pour plating, spread plates, and/or serial dilution if large numbers of organisms are expected. Use proper incubation conditions for aerobic bacteria at 30–35°C for 2 to 5 days; yeasts and molds at 20–25°C for 5 to 7 days and anaerobic bacteria at 30–35°C for 3 to 5 days.

(3) Enumeration of the microorganisms—colony counting is most commonly used.

The two methods used to validate a bioburden recovery method are as follows:

(1) Repetitive recovery involves exposing a single device to sequential extractions and determining the % recovery from the first extraction. This method is appropriate when the bioburden is high and the device is capable of withstanding several extractions. The validation should be performed only once per device or device family after the appropriate extraction fluid and recovery method has been determined. Randomly select a minimum of five (5) similar devices and apply the selected and documented recovery method to each individual device. The total number of organisms recovered from each extraction [there could be as many as four (4) or five (5) extractions] are counted and compared to those recovered in the first extraction by applying the following formula:

$$\% \text{ removal} = \frac{\text{\# cfu recovered from the first extraction}}{\text{total \# cfu recovered from all extractions}}$$

Determine the average recovery, and calculate the correction factor. The correction factor is then applied to each bioburden estimate performed on that device or device family as long as the device and extraction method do not change.

$$\frac{100}{\text{Avg. \% removal}} = \text{Correction factor}$$

An example in Table 12 excerpted from ANSI/AAMI/ISO 11737-1 represents data from five replicates and demonstrates the calculation of correction factors.

From the data, the proportions removed can be calculated as follows:

First treatment	60	50	70	55	45
Total	81	68	84	61	51
% Removal	74	74	83	90	88

Using the mean percentage removal, the correction factor for the recovery efficiency is as follows:

$$\frac{100}{81.2} = 1.22$$

In bioburden estimates determined subsequently using the same extraction method, the mean recoverable number of microorganisms should be multiplied by the calculated correction factor.

(2) Product inoculation involves artificially contaminating a sterile device with a known number of organisms, usually bacterial

TABLE 12. Calculation of Correction Factor.

Treatment	Replicate Count					Mean Colony Count
	1	2	3	4	5	
1	60	50	70	55	45	56
2	10	12	5	2	3	6.4
3	1	0	2	0	0	0.6
4	0	1	0	0	1	0.4
Agar overlay	10	5	7	4	2	5.6
Total colony count	81	68	84	61	51	69

spores, and determining the number removed after exposure to the recovery method. This is appropriate for devices containing low numbers of naturally occurring bioburden. Caution must be used because artificial inoculation may not represent the natural relationship between the normal flora and the device surfaces and material.

Bioburden should be evaluated initially prior to dose verification testing and at least quarterly thereafter prior to or in conjunction with each dose audit validation. Bioburden data should be trended by monitoring the number of organisms and the resistance to ensure control of the device materials and the manufacturing environment. The bioburden recovery method used to recover organisms from product should be validated; especially when the sterilization method employed is radiation. The actual numbers of organisms recovered during testing may not represent the entire organism population actually on the device, but it is the resistance of the bioburden that must be known.

EVALUATION OF BIOBURDEN DATA

Because bioburden numbers are used to select the verification dose during initial validation of any radiation process, an understanding of the effect of bioburden variation is important. Guidance can be found in ISO 11737-3, *Sterilization of medical devices—Microbiological methods—Part 3: Guidance on the evaluation and interpretation of bioburden data.* The most critical variable is the range differential between the highest and lowest recovered number in each group of ten items, especially important being the high value. A bioburden spike is an individual bioburden result, which is two or more times greater than the group average. Because relatively uniform bioburden numbers were used to establish the Table B.1 (from ISO 11137) values, any number falling outside of those values could result in an unexpected result. In some cases, a bioburden spike should be used in setting a dose provided the following criteria are met:

(1) It can be shown with sufficient data that spikes are a consistent and normal part of the device bioburden. It must be evident that spikes are not a rare occurrence indicating a serious problem that would require an investigation.

(2) The spike is within a reasonable range of the average bioburden.

Excessively high spikes can be an indication of a manufacturing/material problem of a lab contaminate. A reasonable range for a spike is usually one that is within a log of the bioburden average.

The recommendation to use bioburden spikes in establishing or verifying sterilization doses is based first on qualifying the spike, as above, and on the following:

(1) The ultimate goal in dose-setting is device safety concerning sterility assurance. Using a spike value may result in a slightly higher sterility assurance level (SAL) for the devices with lower bioburden, but the intended SAL is still being met for the devices, which have spikes.

(2) The use of worst-case situations is a common regulatory practice.

(3) In Method 1 dose-setting procedures, the highest lot average of three is used to set the dose if one lot average is over two times the overall average. The principle of using a spike, if it is over two times the average, is the same.

(4) The use of bioburden spikes was originally incorporated in the ISO 13409 document as a standard practice. Although this section was revised, it was considered an acceptable procedure by most experts involved in microbiology and radiation sterilization.

Examples 1, 2 and 3, excerpted from a presentation by Trabue Bryans (1996) at an AAMI sterilization standards meeting, illustrate how the use of bioburden spikes can avert dose audit failures.

EXAMPLE 1. Product—Lancet (Plastic plus Metal).

Sample #	Batch 1	Batch 2	Batch 3
1	10	3	13
2	2	10	5
3	**39**	24	9
4	9	19	6
5	5	10	11
6	4	7	8
7	**77**	5	10
8	7	**27**	21
9	4	23	4
10	3	12	5
Average	**16**	**14**	**9.2**

- Overall average: 13.1.
- Verification test results: 4 positives = failure.
- Average using spikes: 31.
- Test result using spikes: 1 positive = pass.

EXAMPLE 2. Cotton Gauze Bandage (Large).

Sample #	Batch 1	Batch 2	Batch 3
1	**8900**	3900	1200
2	7700	1200	1800
3	6100	300	4100
4	1100	**16,000**	1100
5	3700	1100	930
6	4100	3400	540
7	8900	1100	**24,000**
8	3600	1200	840
9	**12,000**	270	810
10	1400	690	1100
Average	**5750**	**2916**	**3642**

- **Overall average: 4103.**
- **Verification test results: 15 positives = failure.**
- **Average using spikes: 17,333.**
- **Test result using spikes: 1 positive = pass.**

EXAMPLE 3. Foam Equipment Handle Cover.

Sample #	Batch 1	Batch 2	Batch 3
1	30	110	110
2	75	**2000**	110
3	10	65	80
4	85	270	140
5	**270**	10	170
6	45	280	130
7	15	75	160
8	30	130	70
9	40	40	**340**
10	15	**880**	90
Average	**61.5**	**386**	**140**

- **Overall average: 196.**
- **Verification test results: 6 positives = failure.**
- **Average using spikes: 683.**
- **Test result using spikes: 0 positive = pass.**

BIOBURDEN ISOLATES

A manufacturer may choose to develop information on the radiation resistance of selected isolates recovered from product after exposure to a screening dose, assuming that the isolates' response to radiation is typical of the resistance of that same organism occurring on the product. Conditions of growth of the isolates prior to inoculation onto test samples, their storage on the test samples, and their recovery from the test samples, should be evaluated to ensure comparability.

PRODUCT STERILITY TESTING

Crucial to the validation of any radiation process is product sterility testing of products subjected to sublethal dosing. Guidance for appropriate sterility testing can be found in ANSI/AAMI/ISO 11737-2: 1998, *Sterilization of medical devices—microbiological methods—Part 2: Tests of sterility performed in the validation of a sterilization process.*

There are two (2) general approaches in the performance of product sterility tests. These are as follows:

(1) Direct immersion of the product in growth medium or growth medium into the product followed by incubation for 14 days.
   - The device may be disassembled prior to exposure to facilitate transfer or may be aseptically subdivided prior to transfer to medium container.
   - Sufficient growth media should be used to cover the device or to achieve contact between the growth medium and the whole product.
   - Agitate after placement in growth medium.
   - Maintain contact between medium and product for the duration of the incubation. If the device is large, medium can be swirled daily in order to contact all product surfaces.
(2) Removal of microorganisms from the product by elution and either filtration of or transfer of the removed microorganisms to culture conditions.
   - Use elution techniques similar to those used in bioburden estimation.
   - Addition of a surfactant may be required to improve removal of organisms by moistening the product surfaces.

- Membrane filter should be rated 0.45 microns.
- Aseptically transfer filter to growth medium.

Generally, a single culture medium is used that is optimal for the culturing of aerobic and facultative microorganisms. Soybean-casein digest medium (tryptic soy broth) is commonly used, and the test samples are incubated at 28–32°C for 14 days. Samples should be checked daily for growth and the results recorded. Other commonly used growth media are indicated in Table 13.

The growth medium should be tested for its growth promoting qualities prior to use in any sterility test, and the effects of the product on the ability of microorganisms to grow should be evaluated using the bacteriostasis/fungistasis test. The latter test is performed either before or concurrent with completion of a successful sterility test by adding low numbers of test microorganisms (10 to 100 organisms) to the product/medium container and to medium containers with no product (control) and incubating for an additional 3–5 days. A successful test will result in comparable growth of the test microorganisms in containers with and without product. If the test is negative, it is assumed that some substance in the product has inhibited the growth of the test organisms. The sterility test is also negated and must be repeated after completion of an acceptable bacteriostasis test.

Commonly used growth promotion and bacteriostasis/fungistasis organisms include the following:

- *Candida albicans* for aerobic conditions
- *Bacillus subtilis* for aerobic conditions (facultative organism)
- *Clostridium sporagenes* for anaerobic conditions

TABLE 13. Commonly Used Culture Conditons.

Organism Type	Commonly Used Growth Media	Incubation Temp. °C
Aerobic	Nutrient broth Brain heart infusion broth Soybean-casein digest broth	28 to 32
Fungi	Sabouraud dextrose broth Potato dextrose broth Glucose peptone broth	20 to 25
Facultative	Fluid thioglycolate medium Cooked meat glucose broth	28 to 32

Adapted from ISO 11737-2. 1998.

- *Aspergillus niger* (fungus) for aerobic conditions
- *Micrococcus luteus* for aerobic conditions (grows in the aerobic portion of FTM medium)

If the bacteriostasis/fungistasis test fails, microbiocidal substances can be minimized by:

(1) Addition of neutralizers
(2) Removal of the substance by filtration
(3) Reduction in the concentration of the substance to ineffective levels by dilution, i.e., increase the volume of growth medium or subdivide the product into a number of test containers.

For each product, the following factors that influence the design of the sterility test method should be considered and documented.

(1) The parts(s) of the product for which the sterility claim is made, i.e., sterile fluid pathway only claim means that the internal pathway of the tubing device should be tested by filling with the culture medium.
(2) The physical and/or chemical nature of the product, i.e., if the product is large and bulky, it can be subdivided prior to sterilant exposure, or if the nature of the product indicates that a substance may be released which could adversely affect the number of microorganisms detected, a system to neutralize or remove the substance should be used.
(3) Possible types of contaminating microorganisms and their locations on or within the product

The method for selecting product units for sterility testing during validation can influence the results, so randomly select newly manufactured units from a single batch. Rejected items may be used as long as they were subjected to the same manufacturing environment and conditions. Whenever possible, the entire product unit should be tested. However, if the product is too large or cumbersome, a sample item portion (SIP) can be selected that represents the largest portion of the product unit that can be manipulated. If a SIP is used, it should be prepared and packaged prior to exposure under conditions chosen to minimize alteration of the bioburden.

The occurrence of positive tests during product sterility testing should be investigated to determine if the growth resulted from microorganisms surviving the sterilization process. Any growth should be subcultured and identified, and the organism(s) should be compared to those derived from environmental monitoring or bioburden determinations. The laboratory performing the test should review all procedures and precautions taken as a part of their program to minimize false positives. Examine the lab's false positive rate. The industry average is 0.1%. The lab should indicate if the test sample packaging is compromised in any way prior to testing. If so, the product should not be tested. If there is no indication that a deviation from procedure has occurred during the handling and testing of the device, then the growth must be considered a true positive. Precautions, such as the following, can be taken by the manufacturer to minimize false positives:

- Assure the product sample is small enough to fit within the lab's largest container. The fewer the manipulations required during the test, the better.
- If the product is large and complex, subdivide it in such a manner that the subsequent pieces are easily transferred to the culture medium.
- Transfer test samples after exposure to the sterilization process in a plastic bag to reduce contamination that may accumulate on the outside of the package during shipping.
-

TROUBLESHOOTING MICROBIOLOGICAL FAILURES

Dose audit failures can be costly and result in delays in product distribution and sale. Any investigation to determine a probable cause depends on the data available and a thorough knowledge of the manufacturing process and the test methods used. The following checklist can be used during an investigation to invalidate a failure and allow a reaudit.

Laboratory-related issues include the following:

- Personnel practices—are the operators properly trained, healthy, or fatigued; were appropriate aseptic handling procedures used; was appropriate garb worn and donned in the proper sequence?
- Housekeeping practices—were proper cleaning and decontamination methods used to prepare the test area, were appropriate cleaning agents used for the proper exposure time, was cleaning of all areas performed on schedule?
- Environmental controls—are the temperature and humidity values within specification, was the air pressure differential

maintained continuously, are the HEPA filters certified and working properly, were the variable particulate monitoring results (should evaluate surface and air viables, personnel gloves and gown samples) within established limits, was there any unusual activity in the room or has the room loading increased?

- Sterility testing—does the test laboratory show a pattern of test positives, was the growth media prepared and sterilized properly, are the negative controls contaminated, were test samples handled properly and disinfected before movement into sterility suite, did any unusual events occur before or during the test?
- Product handling—were samples transferred to the lab in plastic bags, was the packaging decontaminated prior to testing, were all packages intact?
- Organisms—identify to the genus and species level, were the identified organisms found in the product bioburden? Or in the sterility suite?

Manufacturing-related issues include the following:

- Manufacturing—have the raw materials or components changed, has there been a process change that could impact bioburden levels, has equipment required maintenance, has there been an increase in equipment numbers or number of personnel working in the room?
- Product samples—were samples properly prepared and packaged; was a SIP used and if so, how was it prepared; was the bioburden distribution considered?
- Irradiation—was the sterilization dose delivered properly?
- Bioburden—were levels higher than historical values, were spikes found in the quarterly audit samples, does the bioburden trending indicate an upward trend, were any positives in the sterility test identified as resistant organisms?

CHAPTER 6

Sterilization Support Testing

IN conjunction with the prevalidation planning activities, an understanding of all of the associated tests required to ensure that the sterile product is safe and effective is critical. The following review will help you decide what test methods to use and when.

SELECTION OF A TEST LABORATORY AND TEST METHODS

A number of important tests will be required to support the validation. These tests can be performed in-house or by an accredited laboratory following industry accepted practice and ISO/ASTM/USP guidelines where applicable. Table 14 lists the required tests and the associated technical reference.

Contract laboratories, like contract sterilizers, are an extension of the manufacturer's operation. As such, the contract test lab must comply with the FDA's QSR rule. Perform an audit to ensure that the lab complies with regulations. The lab should have a quality manual and SOPs describing the test methods. Review the sample control and documentation procedures, the validation of all support equipment, i.e., autoclave, calibration, environmental monitoring and personnel practices in sterility test cleanrooms, media preparation, incubator calibration and control, and training and education of technicians performing the test. Personnel at the test lab can also provide guidance on the appropriate number of samples needed for each type of test requested. The test documentation should reference sample ID, lot number, date sterilized (if sterile), test performed, test method number or description, date performed, technician performing the test and reviewing the test data, the test results, and, in some cases, an indication

59

TABLE 14. Reference Documents for Required Tests.

Reference Document	Test Description
ANSI/AAMI/ISO 11737-1, 11737-3	Bioburden methods
ANSI/AAMI/ISO 11737-2 USP <71>	Sterility—natural product
ISO 11737-2 USP <71>	Bacteriostasis/fungistasis
ANSI/AAMI/ISO 10993-1-12 USP <161>	Biocompatibility—general
CDC Guideline (12/87, 7/91) USP <161> and <85>	LAL test—pyrogen
ANSI/AAMI/ISO 11607 AAMI TIR 22	Functionality—product and packaging
HIMA packaging	Packaging

of whether or not the test results are acceptable. In the case of a sterility failure, the lab should indicate if any deviations from procedure occurred that could explain the failure and should provide a failure investigation report.

ENVIRONMENTAL MONITORING AND CONTROL

Environmental control in areas where terminally sterilized devices are manufactured is a key component in ensuring low levels of product bioburden. Federal Standard 209E contains methods for measuring and quantifying nonviable particulate, and several ISO standards in preparation, ISO 146798 and ISO 14644, will provide methods for evaluating cleanrooms and associated controlled environments. Basically, such variables as airflow, temperature, relative humidity, static electricity, and room pressurization require control within the following ranges:

- airflow velocity: 90–100 ft/min
- temperature: 720°F ± 20°F
- relative humidity: 50% ± 5%
- room pressurization: clean areas should be positive with respect to surrounding areas
- particulate matter: within class limits, if room is classified. For example, a Class 10,000 room should have no more than 10,000 0.5-micron particles per ft^3 of air.

USP XXIV informational chapter <1116> states levels of viable air cleanliness (see the following table). These values are suggested only as guides; each manufacturer must evaluate their own data as part of an overall monitoring program.

Class	cfu/m³ Air	cfu/ft³ Air	cfu/Contact Plate	cfu/Glove	cfu/Personnel Garb
100	<3	<0.1	3 (including floor)	3	5
10,000	<20	<0.5	5 10 (floor)	10	20
100,000	<100	<2.5	ND	ND	ND

ND = not defined.

When a "controlled area" or cleanroom is first installed, a validation should be performed to assess the status of all of the variables mentioned above and to determine if the data derived from sampling supports the proposed room cleanliness level. Develop a sampling plan, which routinely evaluates the above variables, perhaps weekly (in rooms with high activity and use) or monthly (in rooms with low activity and use) depending on the amount of activity in the room. Validate the room "as-built" (with no operations taking place) and during routine operation.

The validation program should be documented by protocol, and the air sampling time intervals (2–3 minutes when particulate count is high >1000; or 5 minutes if particulate level is low <1000) selected should be long enough to provide reproducible numbers. Place the sampling probe for nonviable particulate at table height and in areas where operations are occurring; select several locations in the room in order to assess the cleanliness levels across the room. Sample for viable air particulate using a handheld or table mounted probe in areas where operations are occurring. To support the program, special cleaning and maintenance procedures and operator training must occur.

Microbial contamination can be evaluated by utilizing four (4) sampling and subsequent incubation methods:

(1) Rodac or surface sampling plates: the exposed agar surface is pressed onto the surface of the table, floor, or walls to be moni-

tored and incubated at 30–35°C for 5–7 days. Some plates can be incubated at 20–25°F to better detect molds and fungal organisms. Work surfaces should be selected where operators are working and in areas used infrequently to determine if cleaning procedures are being performed adequately.

(2) Settling plates: the agar surface is exposed to the atmosphere for a selected time period (30 minutes to several hours depending on room cleanliness level) and incubated at 30–35°C for 5–7 days. Plates are placed on surfaces throughout the room and left open for a specified period of time, i.e., during one 8-hour shift or during one sterility-testing shift.

(3) Air samples are taken with a calibrated centrifugal air sampler for a predetermined period of time. Tryptic soy agar strips are used to evaluate bacterial organism and rose bengal agar for molds and fungus. Incubate both at 30–35°C for 5–7 days.

(4) Product bioburden is evaluated by selecting ten random finished device units from lots being manufactured during monitoring activity.

Because cleanroom operations are dynamic processes and identical conditions cannot be duplicated, validation as well as routine testing is performed over time to establish a pattern of control. The technician performing the testing should document all activity occurring in the room, including number of operators, equipment in use, overall activity, amount of packaging material (if any), and location of sampling points. To achieve some consistency, the same locations should be monitored each time during the same shift. This data will be of great value if an investigation is triggered by an unusually high value.

The data should be analyzed statistically, and appropriate action and alert levels should be established. Environmental data have usually been treated by mean + 2 or mean + 3 standard deviations. Three (3) ways review data and identify high clusters, which could signal an out-of-control situation, are plots of values obtained vs. time, histograms, and process control charts. Once enough data has been collected, the action level may be set to equal the 99th percentile of the data, and the alert level may be set to equal the 95th percentile. If the data appears to be a normal distribution, the upper 99th and 95th percentiles may be approximated by the mean +2.326 standard deviations (99th) and by the mean +1.645 standard deviations (95th).

BIOCOMPATIBILITY TESTING

Testing to ensure that irradiated devices are compatible with biological systems is primarily based on the guidelines set forth in ISO 10993-1: *Biological evaluation for medical devices—Part 1: Selection of Tests* (see Table 15). Initially, simple and quick screening tests performed *in vitro* can give valuable information before proceeding to more complicated and costly tests. In all cases, devices radiated at the maximum specified dose should be used in these evaluations.

Cytotoxicity testing is often used as the first step in assessing the biocompatibility of devices and is designed to determine the biological activity of materials on a mammalian cell monolayer. The requirements for this evaluation of devices are defined in ISO 10993-5: *Biological evaluation of devices—Part 5: Tests for cytotoxicity,* in vitro and in *USP XXIV* <87>. The standard cell line is L-929 (ATCC cell line CCL 1, NTCT clone 929) mouse lung fibroblasts.

Three test methods can be used to provide a rapid, sensitive, and inexpensive means of detecting reactivity:

(1) Direct contact method—the test and control samples are applied directly to the cell monolayer in nutrient media. A minimum of 3 cm^2 of surface area (1 cm^2, in triplicate) is required. The monolayers are incubated at 37°C, 5% CO_2 for 24 hours and graded for a zone of reactivity. A rating of moderate or severe results in a test failure.

(2) Agar diffusion method—the test and control samples are applied to a nutrient agar overlay that cushions the cells from mechanical damage. Incubation and scoring are the same as in the direct contact method.

(3) Elution method—an indirect method that uses a fluid extraction of the test samples obtained by placing a known amount of the test and control samples in separate vessels and extracting them under standard conditions. The most common extraction conditions are 24 hours at 37°C. The extract is then applied in triplicate to the cultured cells monolayer and incubated at 37°C, 5% CO_2 for 48 hours. Generally, 0.1 gm elastomer or 0.2 gm of plastic are used for every 1 ml of extracting fluid.

The tests for leachables, such as contaminants, additives, monomers, and degradation products must be conducted by choosing the

TABLE 15. Initial and Supplemental Evaluation Tests for Consideration—FDA-Modified Biocompatibility Matrix—ISO 10993-1.

Device Categories			Biological Tests										
Body Contact		Contact Duration	Short Term								Long-Term		
		A. FDA - Transient (<5 minutes) ISO - Limited (<24 hours) B. FDA Short-Term (5 min - 29 days) ISO - Prolonged (24 hrs - 30 days) C. FDA - Long-Term (≥30 days) ISO - Permanent (>30 days)	Irritation/Intracutaneous Tests	Sensitization Assay	Cytotoxicity	Acute Systemic Toxicity	Hemocompatibility/Hemolysis	Pyrogenicity (Material-Mediated)	Implantation Tests	Mutagenicity (Genotoxicity)	Subchronic Toxicity	Chronic Toxicity	Carcinogenesis Bioassay
External Devices (ISO Surface Devices)	Intact Skin	A	✖	✖	✖								
		B	✖	✖	✖								
		C	✖	✖	✖	▲							
	Mucous Membrane	A	✖	✖	✖	▲							
		B	✖	✖	✖	▲							
		C	✖	✖	✖	▲					○	○	
	Breached or Compromised Surface	A	✖	✖	✖	▲	▲						
		B	✖	✖	✖	▲	▲				▲		
		C	✖	✖	✖	▲	▲			▲	✖	✖	▲
Externally Communicating Devices	Intact Natural Channels/ Tissue	A	✖	✖	✖	▲	▲	▲	▲				
		B	▲	✖	✖	▲	▲	▲	✖	✖	▲		
		C	▲	✖	✖	▲	▲	▲	✖	✖	▲	▲	✖
	Blood Path Indirect	A	✖	✖	✖	▲	✖	▲	▲	▲			
		B	✖	✖	✖	▲	✖	▲	▲	▲	▲		
		C	▲	✖	✖	✖	✖	▲	▲	✖	✖	✖	✖
	Blood Path Direct	A	✖	✖	✖	✖	✖	▲	▲	▲			
		B	✖	✖	✖	✖	✖	▲	▲	✖	▲		
		C	✖	✖	✖	✖	✖	▲	▲	✖	✖	✖	✖

64

TABLE 15. (continued).

Device Categories		Biological Tests											
Body Contact	Contact Duration	Short Term								Long-Term			
	A. FDA - Transient (<5 minutes) ISO - Limited (<24 hours) B. FDA Short-Term (5 min - 29 days) ISO - Prolonged (24 hrs - 30 days) C. FDA - Long-Term (≥ 30 days) ISO - Permanent (>30 days)	Irritation/Intracutaneous Tests	Sensitization Assay	Cytotoxicity	Acute Systemic Toxicity	Hemocompatibility/Hemolysis	Pyrogenicity (Material-Mediated)	Implantation Tests	Mutagenicity (Genotoxicity)	Subchronic Toxicity	Chronic Toxicity	Carcinogenesis Bioassay	

Internal Devices (ISO Implant Devices)														

		Irrit.	Sens.	Cyto.	Acute	Hemo	Pyro	Impl.	Muta.	Subchr.	Chronic	Carcino.
Bone	A	✶	✶	✶	▲	▲	▲	▲	▲			
	B	▲	✶	✶	▲	▲	▲	✶	✶	▲		
	C	▲	✶	✶	▲	▲	▲	✶	✶	▲	✶	✶
Tissue and Tissue Fluids	A	✶	✶	✶	▲	▲	▲	▲	▲			
	B	▲	✶	✶	▲	▲	▲	✶	✶	▲		
	C	▲	✶	✶	▲	▲	▲	✶	✶	▲	✶	✶
Blood	A	✶	✶	✶	✶	✶	▲	✶	▲			
	B	✶	✶	✶	✶	✶	▲	✶	✶	▲		
	C	✶	✶	✶	✶	✶	▲	✶	✶	✶	✶	✶

KEY: ✶ - Tests in both Tripartite and ISO guidelines; ▲ - Tests in Tripartite but *not* in ISO; ○ - Tests in ISO but *not* Tripartite.

N.B. For those devices with possible leachables or degradation products (e.g. absorbable sutures, hemostatic agents, etc.), testing for pharmacokinetics may be required.

Reproductive and development toxicity test may be required for certain materials used for specialized indicators.

Considerations should be given to long-term biological tests where indicated in the table, taking into account the nature and mobility of the ingredients in the materials used to fabricate the device.

appropriate solvent systems that will yield a maximum extraction of the leachable materials. The effects of sterilization on device materials and potential leachables, as well as toxic by-products as a consequence of sterilization should be considered. Additional testing of the device materials and of the final sterilized product or representative samples of the final sterilized product is summarized in Table 16. Different combinations of these procedures using various extracting media make up the USP *in vivo* biological reactivity tests (Class I–VI Plastics Tests).

Other analytical test procedures can provide another means of investigating the biocompatibility of device materials. *In vitro* studies

TABLE 16. ISO/FDA Biocompatibility Testing.

Requirement	Procedure Name
Irritation	USP intracutaneous test*
	Primary skin irritation test
	Primary eye irritation test
	Mucous membrane irritation studies
Sensitization assay	Maximization test (Magnusson/Kligman)
	Patch test (Buehler)
Cytotoxicity	Elution test
	Agar diffusion test
	Direct contact
Acute systemic toxicity	USP systemic toxicity test*
Hemocompatibility/hemolysis	Hemolysis (*in vitro*)
	Thrombogenicity (*in vitro*)
Pyrogenicity	USP LAL pyrogen test
Implantation tests	USP implant test*
	Histopathology on implant sites
Mutagenicity	Ames test
Subchronic toxicity	USP implant test (14–180 days)
	Intravenous toxicity studies (>7 days)
Chronic toxicity	Long-term implant tests
	Lifetime toxicity studies
Carcinogenesis bioassay	Lifetime toxicity studies

*Different combinations of these procedures using various extracting media make up the USP in vitro biological reativity tests (Class I–VI Tests).

of extracts can assess the risks of certain types of *in vivo* reactions. The following analytical chemical tests can provide valuable information:

(1) USP physiochemical test: plastics
(2) USP physiochemical test for elastomeric closures
(3) Extractables from indirect food additives and polymers (21 CFR 177)
(4) Sterilant residues: EtO, ECH, EG
(5) Characterization of metals by atomic absorption spectroscopy
   - extractable metals
   - total metal count
(6) Characterization of organic extractable material
   - ultraviolet/visible spectroscopy
   - gas chromatography
   - liquid chromatography

- protein assay
- infrared spectroscopy

(7) USP purified water monograph

(8) Bulk material characterization

  - infrared spectroscopy—transmission and surface analysis

BACTERIAL ENDOTOXIN AND PYROGEN TESTING

"Microbial pyrogen," as opposed to "gram negative bacterial endotoxin," has become a general descriptive term for many different substances. The pyrogens produced by gram negative bacteria, i.e., the endotoxins, are the ones of significance to the pharmaceutical and medical device industries.

Bacterial endotoxins, found in the outer membrane of gram-negative bacteria are members of a class of phospholipids called lipopolysaccharides (LPS). LPS are not exogenous products of gram negative bacteria. The release of LPS from bacteria takes place after death and lysis of the cell. Good examples of pyrogen producing gram negative bacteria are *Escherichia coli, Proteus, Pseudomonas, Enterobacter,* and *Klebsiella.*

SOURCES

Because endotoxins result from high levels of microorganisms and are not removed by sterilizing or microbiological filters, the subsequent reduction of a high microbiological level will not be associated with a similar reduction of high endotoxin level. As with parenteral drug products, sterile devices have occasionally been shown to be contaminated with endotoxins. Sources have been water, which somehow entered into the manufacturing process. For example, the washing of components such as filter media to be used for the manufacture of filters, or the washing/rinsing of tubing or other plastic devices prior to subsequent sterilization are potential sources of endotoxins.

LAL METHODS

In the medical device industry, LAL testing is performed as a batch release test on products that come into contact with blood or cerebrospinal fluid. Testing is performed on sterile product samples randomly selected from the sterile load. The FDA and USP have recognized the validity of various approaches to using LAL for endotoxin testing.

There are four basic methods commercially available and currently approved by the FDA for end product release testing:

(1) The gel-clot
(2) The turbidimetric (spectrophotometric)
(3) The colorimetric (Lowry protein)
(4) The chromogenic assay

The LAL reagents used in these methods must be obtained from a FDA-registered manufacturer and must be designed specifically for the method chosen. Many of the other LAL methods appearing in the literature are modifications of the gel-clot or turbidimetric test, and some have been designed to use less LAL than the basic method.

Certain products have been known to interfere with the LAL's ability to react with endotoxin. These factors may be chemical or physical. Chemical inhibitors cause chelation of divalent cations necessary for the LAL reaction (i.e., EDTA), protein denaturation (i.e., fluorescein), or pH disruption (i.e., pH outside 6.0–7.5 range). Physical inhibitors include adsorption of endotoxin, or product viscosity. Most will affect all methods although the degree of inhibition may vary. However, most of the inhibition can be overcome by dilution of the product. Other factors such as the shape and type of glassware used in the gel-clot test can also affect the validity of the test. For example, siliconized glassware as well as plastic can inhibit gel-clot formation or prevent accurate spectrophotometric readings of the reaction mixture end point.

Turbidimetric and chromogenic methods cannot be used with certain turbid or colored products. Additionally, precipitate formation, although inhibitory, may be mistaken for a positive response in these methods. One problem associated with the use of the chromogenic method is the formation of a precipitate following the addition of acid to stop color development. Products that require a neutral or basic pH for solubility are most likely to cause this problem.

The necessity of validating the reliability and accuracy of the LAL method for each product tested cannot be overemphasized. Manufacturers can demonstrate this by inoculating the product with low levels of endotoxin and assay for their recovery. The endotoxin concentrations used should be within the lower range of the lysate sensitivity. In addition, several researchers have found that even the selection of lysate reagent source (i.e., the manufacturer of the lysate) can contribute to variability in test results. Therefore, if any change in reagent source is made, the test must be revalidated.

VALIDATION OF THE LAL TEST

(1) Initial qualification of the lab is required to ensure that each analyst can reproducibly perform the test. The following procedures and criteria are used:
   - Gel-clot end point technique—follow guide in USP bacterial endotoxin test monograph.
   - Chromogenic and end point turbidimetric techniques—using the RSE or CSE whose potency is known, assay four replicates of a set of endotoxin concentrations that extend over the labeled linear range. A linear regression analysis is performed on the absorbance values of the standards versus their respective endotoxin concentrations; the coefficient of correlation, r, shall be greater than or equal to 0.980.
   - Kinetic-turbidimetric technique—using the RSE or CSE whose potency, in endotoxin units (EU), is known, assay at least six concentrations in triplicate which extend over the range 0.03–1.0 EU/ml. Perform regression-correlation analysis on the log of the time of reaction (T) versus the log of the endotoxin concentration (E). The coefficient of correlation, r, shall be less than or equal to –0.980.

(2) Inhibition and enhancement testing should be determined for each product before the LAL test is used. All tests should be performed on the appropriate extract dilution. At least three lots of each product type should be tested for inhibition. CDRH recommends two devices for lot size of <30, three devices for lot sizes 30–100, and 3% of lots sized >100, up to a maximum of ten devices per lot.

(3) Routine testing of medical devices—The reference endotoxin is *E. coli* 055:B5 with 0.1 ng/ml the detection limit in the LAL test. *The endotoxin limit for medical devices is 0.5 EU/ml.*
   - Rinse a maximum of ten sterile products per lot with 40 ml of non-pyrogenic water.
   - Prepare endotoxin and set up the endotoxin standard dilution series at least once a day. Endotoxin concentrations of 0.5, 0.25, 0.12, 0.06, and 0.03 EU/ml are common.

- Prepare LAL by reconstitution of lyophilized lysate.
- Set up assay in tubes with product extract, serial dilution of endotoxin bracketing the lysate sensitivity, negative controls (non-pyrogenic water). Add the lysate to each tube, incubate each in a water bath set at 37°C for exactly one hour. Analyze using the method of choice.

There have been several revisions to the analytical procedures outlined in the bacterial endotoxin test since it was first issued in 1980. These changes have enabled the LAL method to be more reliable as a compendial referee test. The significant changes are as follows:

(1) After dilution of endotoxin through a parallel set of solutions, one containing water and the other pH adjusted product, the end point for the reaction mixtures between the two sets should not differ by greater than a twofold difference.
(2) If the product affects the lysate test mixture, then any dilution between the inhibition end point and the MVD can be used.
(3) The maximum a product may be diluted for testing is to be determined using the maximum valid dilution (MVD) formulae. The formula is based upon the product dosage, endotoxin tolerance limit, and the lysate sensitivity. Product dilution beyond this determined factor will render a negative result meaningless. Harmful endotoxin concentrations may be diluted below the detectable range of the lysate.

DEPYROGENATION

It is difficult to remove endotoxins from products once present. It is far better to keep finished products and components relatively endotoxin-free rather than have to remove it once present. The literature cites procedures, such as filtration, irradiation, and ethylene oxide treatment that have limited effect in reducing pyrogen/endotoxin levels. For water for injection (WFI) systems, the two acceptable ways of manufacture are distillation and reverse osmosis (RO). Distillation has been shown to be effective and the most reliable method for removing endotoxin from contaminated water samples. When WFI is produced by RO, the endotoxin level of feed water should be known. Since RO filters are not absolute, it may be necessary to have them in series in order to manufacture pyrogen-free WFI. Whichever system is employed, good practice would include the ability to isolate and evaluate each piece of equipment in a WFI system.

Historically, vials or glass components have been rendered pyrogen-free by dry heat sterilization at high temperatures. Some texts have recommended the depyrogenation of glassware and equipment by heating at a temperature of 250°C for 45 minutes. It has been reported that 650°C for 1 minute or 180°C for 4 hours, likewise, will destroy pyrogens. With respect to manufacturing equipment and transfer lines, depyrogenation by dilution has usually been the method of choice. Utilization of strong alkali or oxidizing solution has occasionally been employed to reduce pyrogens in these storage/delivery systems. However, it should be followed by rinsing with water for injection. Residues in the rinse solution of less than 1 part per million (ppm) can be achieved and have been accepted.

CHAPTER 7

The Validation Protocol

WHETHER you are using a contract sterilizer or in-house equipment, a protocol outlining the procedure that will be used to validate the process must be prepared. The critical first step after validation planning is the protocol. There are many methods and approaches to validation that are scientifically sound, but it has become commonplace for the validation effort to be broken into segments: installation qualification, operational qualification, performance qualification, and requalification. In many cases, each segment is run under its own protocol.

The protocol or written and approved outline of the procedures used to validate the process can take many forms. There are recognized essential elements of a protocol, as defined below. The protocol specifies the validation strategy being used, the product grouping being validated, the bioburden data obtained upon which the verification dose is selected, and the support testing to be performed. The protocol should be reviewed and approved by qualified personnel from the validation team composed of representatives from the quality, engineering, and operations groups prior to initiating the validation (see Appendices 9 and 10 for sample protocols) as well as the quality or validation specialist at the selected contract sterilizer. The protocol should have sufficient details so that there is no misunderstanding about the testing required for performance of a successful validation.

The elements of the protocol are as follows:

- Title page
- Objective/purpose—define the goal of the validation activity. The secret to a successful valuation is a clear definition of the reason the validation is being performed.

73

- Scope—state the range of the project and any history or supportive testing performed prior to initiation of the validation. Here you can elaborate on technical background or rationale used to support your validation process design. State the applicable products, process, or equipment that the validation covers.
- Definitions (if required)—if scientific terms or calculations are used in the text of the protocol that are not commonly understood by all involved parties, define the terms so that all will understand.
- Responsibilities—organize teams and give each team member all of the information needed to understand the scope of their responsibilities in the validation activity. Because concurrent performance of the many steps in the process is critical to success, each team member's role should be well defined.
- Equipment/materials—define the appropriate quality procedures supporting the validation and the equipment and supplies and/or test samples that are required.
- Procedure—outline in detail the steps to be followed. This section of the protocol can be very lengthy and should be segregated into well-defined parts that are easy to follow. Sampling methods and procedures, test methods, and test design should be analytically sound and of appropriate sensitivity.
- Acceptance criteria—define the acceptable ranges and utilize criteria during data analysis to determine the acceptability of the dose experiment. Address deviations by performing a thorough review of the process and test results to determine if the nonconformance invalidates the dose experiment. If a process or test deviation cannot be explained by improper dosing or a test anomaly unrelated to cycle lethality, the experiment should be repeated.
- Requalification—state the dose audit frequency interval; generally quarterly.
- Quarterly dose audit—if a number of dose audits have been performed successfully and trending of the environmental monitoring and bioburden data shows a level of control, then consider a reduction from quarterly to semi-annual audits. A paperwork review by a sterilization specialist should detail these data to support extension of the audit time frame.
- Approvals—obtain appropriate management approval of those individuals of the team responsible for the success of the validation effort.

- References—list all of the relevant ISO standards, AAMI TIRs, and guidelines or other published articles that support the design of the validation.
- Attachments—describe product lines covered by the validation and the selected master challenge product.

CHAPTER 8

Outline of the Sterilization Validation

THE basic requirements and guidance for validation of a radiation sterilization process can be found in ANSI/AAMI/ISO 11137: 1994, *Sterilization of health care products—Requirements for validation and routine control—Radiation sterilization* and in EN 552, *Sterilization of medical devices—Validation and routine control of sterilization by irradiation.*
  The validation process should consist of the following elements:

(1) Product qualification in an irradiator that has been successfully subjected to installation qualification
(2) Installation qualification
(3) Process qualification using a product
(4) Administrative certification to review and approve (1), (2) and (3)
(5) Activities performed to support maintenance of the validation

Figure 11 excerpted from the aforementioned standard, shows a typical validation program.

PRODUCT AND PACKAGING MATERIALS EVALUATION

Following the guidance outlined in Chapter 3, the effects of radiation on the product and packaging materials must be determined. The testing should include an evaluation for the effects of the maximum intended dose on the safety and performance of the product over the shelf life of the product.

77

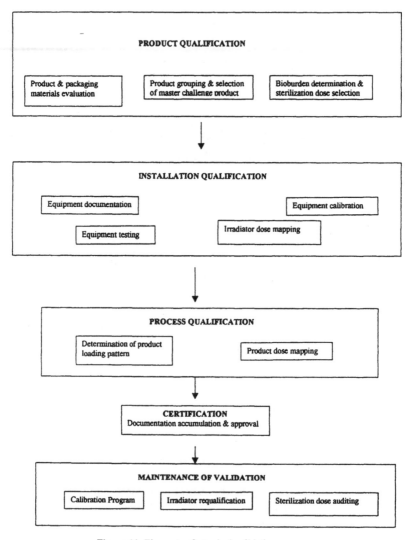

Figure 11 Elements of a typical validation program.

EQUIPMENT QUALIFICATION AND DOCUMENTATION

Documentation should be provided by the contract sterilizer or in-house facility to confirm that the process equipment performs as intended. Process equipment, including the radiation source, conveyor mechanisms, safety devices, and ancillary systems, should be tested to verify satisfactory operation with the design specification. A documented calibration program for gamma irradiators includes irradiation cycle timers or conveyor speed, weighing equipment, and the dosimetry system. For electron beam, the characteristics of the electron beam, the speed of the equipment moving the irradiation containers, weighing equipment, and the dosimetry system should be calibrated. Specifications and procedures should document all aspects of the facility's operations. Documentation should include the following:

- irradiator specifications and characteristics
- description of the location of the irradiator within the premises
- description of the construction and operation of any associated conveyors
- dimensions and description of the materials and construction of irradiation containers
- description of the manner of operation and maintenance of the irradiator and associated conveyor system
- for gamma facilities, dated certificates of source activity and location of individual source capsules within the source frame
- any modification to the irradiator
- calibration of cycle timers or conveyor speed, weighing equipment, and dosimetry systems; characteristics of the electron beam

To transfer a sterilization dose from one type of radiation to another, data should be available to demonstrate the differences in radiation characteristics, particularly radiation energy and the rate at which radiation is delivered, do not affect the microbiocidal effectiveness. Such studies are *not* required for transfer in the following situations:

(1) Between one gamma radiation facility to another gamma radiation facility
(2) Between one electron beam radiant facility to another electron beam radiant facility using equivalent operating conditions

STERILIZATION DOSE SELECTION

The methods of selection of the sterilization dose rely on data derived from the inactivation of the microbial population in its natural state and are based on a probability model for the inactivation of microbial populations. The selection depends upon experimental verifi-

TABLE 17. Standard Distribution of Resistance (SDR) D_{10} Values
(Tallentire, 1998).

D_{10} kGy	1	1.5	2	2.5	2.8
Probability	0.65487	0.22493	0.06302	0.03179	0.01213
D_{10} kGy	3.1	3.4	3.7	4	4.2
Probability	0.00786	0.0035	0.00111	0.00072	0.00007

cation that the response to radiation of the product bioburden is greater than that of a microbial population having a standard resistance. Using computational methods and the standard distribution of resistances shown in Table 17, individual doses required to achieve stipulated SALs have been calculated for levels of bioburden on product just prior to irradiation. These values are the basis of the dose table included in Appendix 10 (use after approval of ISO 11137 revision).

The basis for Method 1 is the contention that the model population presents a more severe challenge (worse case) to the radiation sterilization process than the natural microflora normally present on or in products to be sterilized; this population is referred to as Population C. If a more precise sterilization dose is required, then Method 2 can be applied. If the bioburden population is low and easy to sterilize and the device materials are sensitive to irradiation, then a lower sterilization dose can be validated (see Figure 12).

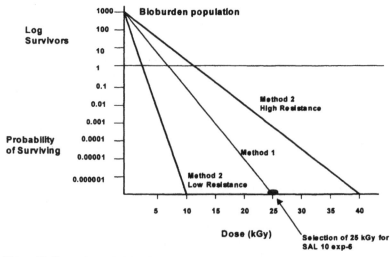

Figure 12 Comparison of bioburden-based validation techniques for radiation sterilization (adapted from AAMI ST 69).

The substantiation of 25 kGy approach using the VD_{max} method is the outcome of research prompted by the occurrence of unexpected failures of verification dose experiments using methods outlined in ISO TR13409, particularly for products with low bioburden. It is based on Population C but recognizes the two-phase nature of the survival curve demonstrated in dose setting applications using Method 1. The upper slope (D_{10}) of the curve from the initial bioburden level to the SAL level of 10^{-2} is the primary D_{10} (PD_{10}), and the slope of the curve from this point to the 10^{-6} SAL level is the terminal D_{10} (TD_{10}) as shown in Figure 13. For a bioburden level in the range of 1 to 50, the D_{10} value approximates the theoretical linear survival curve, whereas in the range of 51 to 1000, the D_{10} value was TD_{10}. The verification dose at a 10^{-1} SAL (instead of 10^{-2}) is used. This method preserves the conservative nature of Method 1 and depends upon experimental verification that the response of the bioburden to radiation is greater (less resistant) than that of Population C.

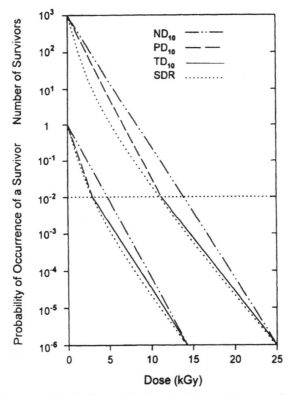

Figure 13 Responses defined by D_{lin} and TD_{10} for each of the population sizes of 1 and 1000.

Four approaches to selecting of the dose can be used depending on the batch size and device bioburden level (Table 18):

(1) Method 1: determination of the bioburden which is then used to select and test a 10^{-2} verification dose based on Population C
(2) Methods 2A and 2B: incremental dosing of device samples
(3) Method VD_{max}: substantiation of 25 kGy as a sterilization dose; appropriate for devices with <1000 cfu/device. (New method is in draft form at publication. It will become the preferred method for substantiation of 25 kGy in the revision of ISO 11137.)

Recent reexamination of dose setting methods shows that Method 1 is generally a reliable and safe method of dose setting; although it tends to be less discriminating with small population sizes. Information for proper bioburden determination should be obtained from competent microbiological laboratory services following guidance in accordance with ISO 11737, Parts 1, 2, 3 as outlined in Chapter 5.

DOSE SETTING USING METHOD 1 (BIOBURDEN METHOD)

This method depends upon experimental verification that the response to radiation of the product bioburden is equal to or less than that based on historical data of microbial population having a standard resistance. In other words, the probability model used to develop Table B.1 (designation of this table will change in the revision of ISO 11137 under way at the time of publication) assumes that the in situ

TABLE 18. Comparison of the Dose Setting Methods.

	Method 1	Method 2 A and B	VD_{max} 25kGy
Rationale	Estimate dose for SAL = 10^{-2}, extrapolate to required SAL	Determine dose by incremental dosing, calculate dose required for SAL	Assume 25 kGy produces SAL = 10^{-6}
Production lot size	All	Medium-Large	All
Production rate	Any	Frequent	Any
Bioburden limit	1,000,000	None	≤1000
Samples for testing	130 units	Method 2A-840 Method 2B-780 (200 can be returned to inventory)	40

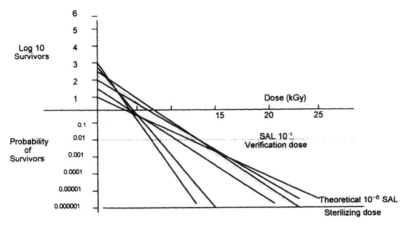

Figure 14 Method 1 population (1000 cfu).

bioburden is a mixture of homogeneous populations, each having its own unique susceptibility to radiation and its own rate of inactivation (see Figure 14), which presents a lesser challenge than the model. Testing is performed at a dose calculated to give a sterility assurance level of 10^{-2}. This is called the verification dose and represents the probability that one unit of product out of 100 units contains one or more viable organisms. Therefore, sterility testing of products subjected to the verification dose should produce 1% positives. If a larger than expected number of units test positive, then either the resistance of the bioburden is higher than expected or the bioburden has been underestimated. Method 1 is preferred in most situations because of its reasonable cost and study time. Sample requirements initially total 136 (100 for the dose experiment, 30 for bioburden determination and six for bacteriostasis/fungistasis testing) and 110 (100 for the dose experiment and 10 for bioburden determination) thereafter on each quarterly dose audit.

The sequence of steps required to validate a radiation process using Method 1 is summarized in Appendices 1 and 2 and outlined here as follows:

(1) Select the appropriate SAL and obtain samples of product units.
(2) Determine the bioburden levels using ten final packaged products from three different batches. Apply a correction factor before selecting the verification dose. If a SIP is to be used, determine the appropriateness of the SIP (Chapter 4). Even though validation of the bioburden recovery method is not required, it is recommended

in order to have a better understanding of the actual numbers of organisms that will be subjected to the verification dose.

(3) Determine the batch average of each of the three batches. Be sure to take into account any "spikes" (see page 51).

(4) Calculate the overall batch average.

(5) Select the verification dose from the dose table using either the highest batch average (if one or more batch averages are greater than the overall batch average) or the overall batch average. If spikes are present, use spike values (or spike averages) in place of the batch average.

(6) Perform the verification dose using 100 final packaged products or SIPs from a single batch. The samples can be selected from any of the three batches from which the bioburden samples were taken or from a fourth batch. Send the packaged samples to the irradiator and indicate the purpose and the dose. The actual dose delivered can vary by +10%. If the dose does not meet the specification, do not proceed to the sterility test. Repeat the verification dose using fresh samples.

(7) Sterility test the 100 units. Bacteriostasis/fungistasis testing should also be performed if this is the first time the product has been subjected to a sterility test.

(8) Review results to assess the acceptability of the experiments:
   - 1 or 2 positive tests = acceptable
   - >2 positives with no deviations in the testing or dose delivery = dose method is not valid for the product and the alternative method should be used (Method 2)

(9) Establish sterilization dose if test is acceptable by finding the closest bioburden number in the dose table equal to or greater than the average bioburden and the selected SAL level.

METHOD 1 AUDIT

A review of the environmental monitoring data and manufacturing controls, together with the bioburden estimate data, should be conducted in conjunction with each audit. One hundred ten test samples are selected randomly from a single batch; ten are tested for bioburden and 100 are dosed at the original verification dose. Sterility test results should be evaluated as follows:

(1) If two or fewer positives are obtained, the original dose is acceptable.

(2) If 3–4 positives are obtained, the original sterilization dose might not be acceptable and should be augmented immediately. A retest using 100 product units at the same verification dose may be performed to determine if the augmented dose is to continue.

- If, on retest, two or fewer positives are obtained and the environmental and bioburden data indicate no values outside specification, use of the original dose may be resumed.
- If, on retest, 3–4 positives are obtained, follow audits actions under 5–6 positives.
- If, on retest, 5 or more positives are obtained, follow steps under 7 or more positives.
- If augmentation of the dose is continued, the next quarterly audit should be conducted using the revised verification dose. If augmentation of the sterilization dose is not continued, the next quarterly audit is conducted using the original verification dose. A repeat of the sterilization dose audit is *not* permitted unless there is documented evidence that the audit was invalidated by unacceptable performance of a test procedure (i.e., sterility test) or due to low dosing.

(3) If 5–6 positives are obtained, the original doses are not adequate and should be augmented immediately, and a retest is not allowed. At the next quarterly audit, the revised verification dose should be used or when the sterilization dose has been reestablished, the new verification dose.

(4) If 7 or more positives are obtained and there is no significant increase in the bioburden estimate, it is assumed that the bioburden resistance is changed and the sterilization dose cannot be augmented and should be reestablished.

DOSE AUGMENTATION FOR METHOD 1

A revision of the verification dose and an augmentation can be carried out if the following conditions are present during the audit procedure (see a worked example in Appendix 8):

(1) 3–4 positives occur
(2) 5–6 positives occur and the bioburden shows an increase
- Change the verification and sterilization dose to the greater values utilizing a bioburden estimate obtained on audit or by multiplying the average bioburden estimate by a factor of 10

and using the new value to obtain the new verification dose from the dose table.

(3) if 5–6 positives occur during audit and the bioburden shows no increase, the sterilization dose cannot be augmented. The sterilization dose shall be reestablished.

VALIDATION USING METHOD 2

Method 2 is less attractive because of the large number of test samples required as well as the higher cost of subjecting samples to multiple sublethal doses (minimum of nine for Method 2A) needed to quantify the radiation resistance of the actual bioburden. This process can, however, yield a final sterilization dose lower than Method 1 because the dose is based on a conceivably less resistant bioburden than the resistant organisms in the model population (SDR) used as the basis of the dose table used in Method 1. As many as 640 product samples for Method 2A could be required. Product units from each of three production lots are exposed to incremental radiation doses, starting at 2 kGy, then increasing in 2 kGy increments, i.e., 4 kGy and 6 kGy. The products are then sterility tested to determine a verification dose expected to yield a SAL of 10^{-2} (1% positives). The results of the sterility test are used to make an estimate of the D_{10} value, and this estimate is used for extrapolation to SALs below 10^{-2}.

Two procedures are available for validation of Method 2: Method 2A for products with bioburden as would be expected from normal manufacturing processes and Method 2B for products with a consistent and very low bioburden. Method 2B requires that the entire product unit (SIP = 1) be used, while Method 2A may be used for either an entire product unit or a portion thereof (SIP ≤ 1.0).

METHOD 2A VALIDATION

Formulas used in calculations can be found in ISO 11137.

(1) Select SAL and obtain product samples.
(2) Select 280 product samples randomly from each of three production lots.
(3) Perform incremental dose experiments irradiating twenty product units from each of three lots at one of a series of not less than nine doses, increasing in 2 kGy increments. The delivered doses can vary from the nominal dose ±1.0 kGy or ±10%.

(4) Sterility test the product units at 30°C ±2° for 14 days. Record the number of positive and negative tests.

(5) For each of the three lots, determine the lowest dose (FFP kGy) where at least one of the twenty tests is negative. Find the median value. Determine A kGy from Table B.2 (from ISO 11137) using the number of positive sterility tests at the median FFP kGy dose.

(6) For each of the three lots, determine the d^* kGy by either finding the lowest dose of two consecutive doses at which all tests are negative, followed by no more than one further positive test, or by finding the lowest dose at which one positive in twenty tests occurs, immediately preceded and followed by incremental doses at which all tests are negative.

(7) Designate the D kGy if the highest lot d^* kGy exceeds the median lot d^* kGy by less than 5 kGy, the median batch d^* kGy becomes the D^* kGy, or if the highest lot d^* kGy exceeds the median lot d^* Gy by 5 kGy or more, the highest lot d^* kGy becomes the D^* kGy.

(8) Establish the lot in which the d^* kGy equals the D^* kGy and designate it the CD^* lot.

(9) Perform the verification dose experiments by irradiating 100 products from the CD^* lot at a dose of D^* kGy. Designate the delivered dose as DD^* kGy. The actual dose may vary by +1.0 kGy or +10%, whichever is greater. If the delivered dose is less than 90% of the DD^* kGy dose, the test may be repeated.

(10) Test the irradiated products at 30°C ±2° for 14 days.

(11) Evaluate the test results by finding the first no positives (FNP) kGy as follows:
- If CD^* is 2 or less, FNP kGy is equal to DD^* kGy.
- If CD^* is greater than 2 but less than 10, FNP kGy = DD^* kGy + 2.0 kGy.
- If CD^* is greater than 9 and less than 16, FNP kGy = DD^* kGy + 4.0 kGy.
- If CD^* is greater than 15, D^* kGy should be redetermined.

(12) Establish the DS kGy (dose required to inactivate 90% of the organisms surviving D^{**} kGy) from FFP kGy and FNP kGy using the following:
- When (FNP − FFP) < 10 kGy, then DS kGy = 2 + 0.2 (FNP − FFP) kGy.

- When (FNP − FFP) is > 10 kGy, then DS kGy = 0.4 + (FNP − FFP) kGy.

(13) Establish D^{**} kGy = DD^* kGy + [log (CD^*)] (DS) kGy

(14) Calculate sterilization dose:
- Sterilization dose = D^{**} kGy + [−log (SAL) − log (SIP) − 2] $(DS$ kGy).
- D^{**} kGy is the estimate of the dose that will provide a 10^{-2} SAL for the test samples.
- DS kGy is an estimate of the dose required to inactivate 90% of the organisms surviving the 10^{-2} verification dose $(D^{**}$ kGy).

METHOD 2A AUDIT

Once the sterilization dose has been established, periodically irradiate 100 product units at the dose used to establish the 10^{-2} SAL (the verification dose of D^{**} kGy), and perform subsequent sterility testing. The procedure is as follows:

(1) Randomly select 110 product units.
(2) Use the same SIP and bioburden methods to determine bioburden.
(3) Irradiate 100 product units at the verification dose found in the original dose setting experiment $(D^{**}$ kGy). The actual dose may vary by +10%.
(4) Perform the sterility test.
(5) Evaluate the results as follows:
- If ≤2 positives are obtained, the original sterilization dose is acceptable.
- If 3–4 positives are obtained, the original dose may not be acceptable. The dose shall be augmented immediately as defined under Method 1 dose augmentation. A retest at the original verification dose may be performed to determine if augmentation must continue. If ≤2 positives are obtained and the bioburden and environmental monitoring show no high values, use of the original sterilization dose may be resumed.
- If 5–6 positives are obtained, the original sterilization dose is not adequate. The sterilization dose shall be augmented immediately.
- If >7 positives are obtained and there is a change to the

upside in the bioburden, the sterilization dose cannot be augmented and must be reestablished.

METHOD 2B VALIDATION

The steps are similar to Method 2A, but the incremental dosing units increase in 1 kGy increments instead of 2 kGy.

(1) Select SAL and obtain product samples.

(2) Select 260 product samples randomly from each of the three production lots. The whole product unit is used (SIP = 1).

(3) Perform incremental dose experiments irradiating twenty product units from each of the three lots at one of a series of not less than eight doses, starting at 1 kGy and increasing in 1 kGy increments. The delivered doses can vary from the nominal dose ±0.5 kGy or ±10%. At 1 kGy the dose may vary by only ±0.2 kGy.

(4) Sterility test the product units at 30°C ±20 for 14 days. Record the number of positive and negative tests. The number of sterility test positives should not exceed 14+/20 at any dose.

(5) For each of the three lots, determine the lowest dose (ffp kGy) where at least one of the twenty tests is negative. Find the median value. Determine A kGy from Table B.3 (from ISO 11137) using the number of positive sterility tests at the median ffp kGy dose.

$$A \text{ kGy} = (1 \text{ kGy}) \frac{(\log\ 10(\log_e 20) - \log\ 10[\log_e(20/n)])}{(\log\ 10(\log_e 20) - \log\ 10[\log_e(20/19)])}$$

Calculate FFP kGy = median ffp dose − A kGy

(6) For each of the three lots, determine the d^* kGy by either finding the lowest dose of two consecutive doses at which all tests are negative, followed by no more than one further positive test, or by finding the lowest dose at which one positive in twenty tests occurs, immediately preceded and followed by an incremental dose at which all tests are negative.

(7) Designate the D^* kGy if the highest lot d^* kGy exceeds the median lot d^* kGy by less than 5 kGy, the median batch d^* kGy becomes the D^* kGy, or if the highest lot d^* kGy exceeds the

median lot d^* Gy by 5 kGy or more, the highest lot d^* kGy becomes the D^* kGy.

(8) Establish the lot at which the d^* kGy equals the D^* kGy and designate it the CD^* lot.

(9) Perform the verification dose experiments by irradiating 100 products from the CD^* lot at a dose of D^* kGy. Designate the delivered dose as DD^* kGy. The actual dose may vary by +1.0 kGy or +10%, whichever is greater. If the delivered dose is less than 90% of the DD^* kGy dose, the test may be repeated.

(10) Test the irradiated products at 30°C ±2° for 14 days. Designate the number of positive tests as CD^*.

(11) Evaluate the test results by finding the first no positives (FNP) kGy as follows:

- If CD^* is 2 or less, FNP kGy is equal to DD^* kGy.
- If CD^* is greater than 2 but less than 10, FNP kGy = DD^* kGy + 2.0 kGy.
- If CD^* is greater than 9 and less than 16, FNP kGy = DD^* kGy + 4.0 kGy.
- If CD^* is greater than 15, D^* kGy should be redetermined.

(12) Establish the DS kGy (dose required to inactivate 90% of the organisms surviving D^{**} kGy) from FFP kGy and FNP kGy using the following:

$$DS \text{ kGy} = 1.6 + 0.2 \, (\text{FNP} - \text{FFP}) \text{ kGy},$$

$$\text{if (FNP} - \text{FFP) is} < 0, \text{ set FNP} - \text{FFP} = 0$$

(13) Establish D^{**} kGy = DD^* kGy + [log (CD^*)] (DS) kGy.

(14) Calculate sterilization dose:

- Sterilization dose = D^{**} kGy + [−log (SAL) − log (SIP) − 2] (DS) kGy.
- D^{**} kGy = estimate of the dose that will provide a 10^{-2} SAL for the test samples.
- DS kGy is an estimate of the dose required to inactivate 90% of the organisms surviving the 10^{-2} verification dose (D^{**} kGy).

METHOD 2B DOSE AUDIT

Auditing on a quarterly basis is performed by irradiating 100 product units at the dose used to establish the 10^{-2} SAL (D^{**} kGy). The method is the same as outlined in the Method 2A audit.

METHOD 2A AND 2B DOSE AUGMENTATION

Revision of the verification dose and augmentation of the sterilization dose occurs when

(1) Three or four positives occur.
(2) Five or six positives occur and the bioburden shows an increase.

Use the following equation to calculate the revision verification dose for both methods:

$$D^{**} \text{ kGy} = DD^* \text{ kGy} + [\log (CD^*)](DS) \text{ kGy}$$

Augmented sterilization dose for Method 2A:

$$\text{Sterilization dose} = $$
$$D^{**} \text{ kGy} + (-\log (\text{SAL}) - \log (\text{SIP}) - 2)(DS) \text{ kGy}$$

Augmented sterilization dose for Method 2B:

$$\text{Sterilization dose} = D^{**} \text{ kGy} + [-\log (\text{SAL}) - 2)](DS) \text{ kGy}$$

where CD^* is the number of positive sterility tests from exposure to the audit dose and DS kGy is calculated using the equation in step 12. See worked examples in the ISO 11137 standard.

METHOD VD_{max} SUBSTANTIATION OF 25 kGy DOSE

This method (which will replace TR 13409 upon revision of ISO 11137), based on the SDR of Method 1, can be used for production batches of any size with an average bioburden of less than 1000 cfu per device. The method preserves the conservative aspects of the resistance characteristics of the SDR, but is more accurate for low bioburden products.

The following steps are included in this method (a worked example is included in Appendix 7)

(1) Obtain at least ten product units from each of three production batches immediately prior to sterilization.

(2) Determine the average bioburden on each product as outlined in ISO 11737-1 and average the bioburden values for each batch. Apply the correction factor based on the validation of bioburden recovery. Compare the three batch averages and select the grand average or one average if two or more times the overall average.

(3) Establish the verification dose using Table 19 [Table 2 in AAMI TIR (draft), *Sterilization of health care products—Radiation sterilization—Substantiation of 25 kGy as a sterilization dose*]. For SIP =1 find the closest bioburden value greater than or equal to the average. For SIP < 1 calculate the bioburden of a SIP = 1 by dividing the SIP bioburden by the SIP decimal value. Using the closest bioburden value, locate the SIP dose reduction factor and use it in the following equation to find the SIP verification dose for ten samples.

SIP Verification Dose = (SIP = 1 Verification Dose)

+ (log SIP * SIP Dose Reduction Factor)

(4) Perform the verification dose experiment by selecting ten product units from a single batch. These may be selected from any one of the bioburden batches or a fourth batch. Irradiate the product units at the verification dose. The actual dose may vary from the calculated dose by not more than +10%. If the delivered dose is less than 90% of the verification dose, the experiment may be repeated.

(5) Sterility test the product units according to ISO 11737-2 using soybein-casein digest broth incubated at 30°C ±2°C for 14 days. Record the number of positive tests.

(6) Interpretation of results. If no more than one positive test is observed in the 10 tests, 25 kGy is substantiated as the sterilization dose to achieve at least a 10^{-6} SAL. If 2+/10 tests are observed, a confirmatory verification dose experiment shall be conducted. If 3+/10 tests are observed, 25 kGy is *not* substantiated, and another dose setting method must be used.

(7) Confirmatory verification dose experiment (if required): randomly select ten product units from a single batch (can be from the batches previously sampled or from a new batch). Use the same dose as determined initially, and irradiate the ten product units at the confirmatory verification dose. The same dose tolerances apply. Sterility testing results are evaluated as follows:

TABLE 19. Verification and Sterilization Dose Selection for VD_{max}.

Bioburden	Verification Dose kGy	SIP Factor	Augmentation Value kGy
1	4.2	4.17	4.2
2	5.2	3.97	4.0
3	5.7	3.86	3.9
4	6.1	3.79	3.8
5	6.3	3.73	3.7
6	6.6	3.69	3.7
7	6.7	3.65	3.7
8	6.9	3.62	3.6
9	7.0	3.59	3.6
10	7.1	3.57	3.6
11	7.2	3.55	3.6
12	7.3	3.53	3.5
13	7.4	3.51	3.5
14	7.5	3.50	3.5
15	7.6	3.48	3.5
16	7.6	3.47	3.5
17	7.7	3.46	3.5
18	7.8	3.45	3.4
19	7.8	3.43	3.4
20	7.9	3.42	3.4
22	8.0	3.40	3.4
24	8.1	3.39	3.4
26	8.1	3.37	3.4
28	8.2	3.36	3.4
30	8.3	3.34	3.3
35	8.4	3.31	3.3
40	8.6	3.29	3.3
45	8.7	3.27	3.3
50	8.8	3.25	3.2
55	8.9	3.23	3.2
60	8.9	3.21	3.2
65	9.0	3.20	3.2
70	9.1	3.19	3.2
75	9.1	3.17	3.2
80	9.2	3.15	3.2
85	9.1	3.11	3.2
90	9.1	3.08	3.2
95	9.1	3.05	3.2
100	9.0	3.01	3.2
110	9.0	2.96	3.2
120	9.0	2.91	3.2
130	8.9	2.86	3.2
140	8.9	2.83	3.2
150	8.9	2.79	3.2
160	8.8	2.76	3.2
170	8.8	2.72	3.2
180	8.8	2.69	3.2
190	8.7	2.67	3.3

(continued)

TABLE 19. (continued).

Bioburden	Verification Dose kGy	SIP Factor	Augmentation Value kGy
200	8.7	2.64	3.3
220	8.7	2.60	3.3
240	8.6	2.56	3.3
260	8.6	2.52	3.3
280	8.6	2.49	3.3
300	8.6	2.46	3.3
325	8.5	2.43	3.3
350	8.5	2.40	3.3
375	8.5	2.37	3.3
400	8.4	2.34	3.3
425	8.4	2.32	3.3
450	8.4	2.30	3.3
475	8.4	2.28	3.3
500	8.4	2.26	3.3
525	8.3	2.24	3.3
550	8.3	2.22	3.3
575	8.3	2.21	3.3
600	8.3	2.19	3.3
650	8.3	2.16	3.4
700	8.2	2.14	3.4
750	8.2	2.12	3.4
800	8.2	2.09	3.4
850	8.2	2.07	3.4
900	8.1	2.05	3.4
950	8.1	2.04	3.4
1000	8.1	2.02	3.4

- 0+/10 (total of 2+/20) – 25 kGy is substantiated.
- 1-10+/10 (total of >3/20) – 25 kGy is not substantiated.

DOSE AUDIT

A dose audit for product in regular production shall be performed once per quarter in order to detect changes in the bioburden as follows:

(1) Obtain a random sample of twenty product units from a single production batch.
(2) Determine bioburden on ten products.
(3) Perform dose audit experiment using the dose from the original dose experiment and ten product units.
(4) Sterility test the product.
   - If 1+/10, 25 kGy is substantiated.

- If 2+/10, the confirmatory verification dose experiment is conducted.
- If 3+ or more, 25 kGy is not substantiated, and the 25 kGy shall be immediately augmented and a dose setting method employed.

(5) Confirmatory dose audit experiment, if required, is performed using ten product units, irradiated at verification dose and sterility tested.
- If 0+/10, 25 kGy is substantiated.
- If 1+/10 or more, 25 kGy is not substantiated. The 25 kGy dose shall be immediately augmented and a dose setting method employed.

DOSE AUGMENTATION

When three or more sterility test positives are observed in the dose audit experiment, augment the dose using the average bioburden and Table 2 from AAMI TIR, find the closest bioburden value equal to or greater than the average bioburden value, and read across the table to the Dose Augmentation Value column. Use this value in the following equation to calculate the augmented sterilization dose:

Augmented dose (kGy) = 25 kGy + dose augmentation value

SELECTION OF A STERILIZATION DOSE
FOR A SINGLE PRODUCTION BATCH

This method is applicable only for validation of a sterilization dose for a single production batch as outlined in AAMI TIR 15844, *Sterilization of health care products—Radiation sterilization—Selection of a sterilization dose for a single production batch.* The estimate of the bioburden is made on the batch, and the verification experiment and sterilization dose selection is consistent with ISO 11137, Method 1.

The following procedural steps will validate the appropriate sterilization dose (a worked example is shown in Appendix 8):

(1) Select the SAL and obtain a sample of ten product units selected randomly from the batch.
(2) Determine the average bioburden.

(3) Establish the verification dose based on the average bioburden and Table 2 of the AAMI TIR 15844.

(4) Perform the verification dose experiment by randomly selecting 100 product units (or SIPs) from the entire batch. Irradiate the products at the verification dose. The delivered dose can differ from the calculated dose by +10%. Subject the irradiated units to a sterility test. Incubate in soybean-casein digest broth at 28–32°C for 14 days. Remember to perform bacteriostasis/fungistasis testing if this test product has not been evaluated before.

(5) Review test results.
- Two or fewer positive tests are acceptable.
- If more than two positives result, this method of dose setting is not valid, and an alternate dose selection method should be used unless the result can be ascribed to estimation of the bioburden, use of the average bioburden = value, the performance of the sterility test of the dose delivery.

(6) Establish the sterilization dose using Table 2 in the AAMI TIR 15844.

ALTERNATE SAMPLING PLANS FOR DOSE VERIFICATION AND AUDIT

A reduction of the number of products used for quarterly dose audits may be desirable if it can be accomplished while maintaining assurance of the desired SAL. Phillips has shown that it is possible to replace the simple random sampling plan outlined in ISO 11137 as Method 1 with a double random sample (Table 20). The first random sample of fifty-two units is dosed and sterility tested with an accept number of 0 positives, and the second random sample, if the first failed, of fifty-two units with a combined (104) accept number of 2 positives.

To perform an alternative sampling plan from the table row indicated with an *, follow these steps:

(1) Select fifty-two products (or product SIP) from a single batch.

(2) Irradiate the product at the verification dose derived from the method 1 dose table. The actual dose may vary by not more than +10%.

(3) Sterility test each product.

TABLE 20. Summary of Sampling Plans and Sampling Schemes (from AAMI TIR 15483).

Application	Table # Method	Test Sample Size	Accepts # Pos./ # Tested	Retest # Pos./ # Tested	Fail # Pos./ # Tested	Retest Sample Size	Accept Total # Pos./ Total # Tested	Fail Total # Pos./ Total # Tested
Method 1 Dose	Table 1 ISO 11137	100	≤2/100	NA	≥3/100	NA	NA	NA
Verification*	Table 2 Alternative	52	0/52	1-2/52	≥3/52	52	≤2/104	≥3/104
Method 1 and 2	Table 3 ISO 11137	100	≤2/100	3-4/100	>7/100	100	≤2/100	≥5/100
Sterilization	Table 4 alternative	50	0/50	1-3/50	≥4/50	100	≤4/150	≥5/150
Dose	Table 5 alternative	70	≤1/70	2-5/70	≥6/70	130	≤5/200	≥6/200
Audit	Table 6 alternative	140	≤4/140	NA	≥5/140	NA	NA	NA
Method 1 Verification	Table 7 Part 1 QSS tightened	60	0/60	1-2/60	≥3/60	60	≤2/120	≥3/120
Sterilization Dose Audit	Table 8 Part 2 QSS reduced	35	0/35	1-2/35	≥4/35	110	≤4/145	>5/145

97

(4) Interpret the results.
- If no positives, experiment is acceptable, and sterilization dose can be determined from the Method 1 dose table.
- If 1–2 positives, select either from the original batch or another batch an additional fifty-two products; irradiate and sterility test. Sum the number of positive tests from the first and second sets. If the total is not more than 2 positive tests, the experiment is acceptable.
- If more than 3 positives and their occurrence cannot be attributed to incorrect bioburden, sterility testing, or delivery of the verification dose, this method of dose setting is not valid. Augmentation cannot be performed.

CHAPTER 9

Final Report

THE final report is a compilation of all of the data, including dose maps, certification of verification and sterilization dose, bioburden and sterility test reports that support the successful completion of the validation. Generally, the report is organized in a notebook and contains the approved and signed protocol, all data and test reports from the dose verification experiment, and the approved and signed final report. The sections of the final report are as follows:

- Title page
- Purpose: state what the report contains or what validation has been successfully completed.
- Scope: state the range of the project and any history or supportive testing performed prior to initiation of the validation.
- Responsibilities: define in the protocol and do not repeat in the report.
- Equipment/materials: define in the protocol and do not repeat in the report unless additional supplies and equipment were used.
- Procedure: outline in detail the steps that were followed. If any deviations occurred, be sure to discuss them and the results. If changes to the protocol were required during the validation, the approved and signed Addendum should be included in the report.
- Results: discuss the results from the dose verification experiment and determine if the results comply with the acceptance criteria defined in the protocol. Any rationale used to repeat the experiment or augment the dose must be documented.
- Conclusion: state whether the data met the acceptance criteria. Discuss any deviations and any rationale for rejecting any dose experiments or test results.

- Requalification: define the time frame for revalidation of the process; the industry standard is quarterly. If acceptable dose audits have been performed for one year and the bioburden is in control, the audit frequency interval can be increased to every six months.
- Approvals: obtain appropriate management approval of those individuals on the team responsible for the success of the validation effort.
- Attachments: provide a copy of the radiation certification, and bioburden and sterility test data.

CHAPTER 10

Routine Monitoring and Control

AFTER successful completion of the sterilization validation, a process specification must be written that explains the proper procedures to be followed routinely. The process specification must describe the aspects of the sterilization process necessary to assure conformance with the validated dose and dose mapping and must be maintained with an established change control procedure. All specified process parameter values must be met or product cannot be released as sterile. The process specification should include the following:

(1) Identity of radiation modality qualified for sterilization
(2) List of the items approved for sterilization in the process covered by the specification, i.e., the product listing
(3) The maximum dose allowed and the sterilization dose
(4) Written procedures for sterilization process operations or reference to specific operator manuals
(5) Sterilizer tote loading configurations and dose mapping showing the relationships between the reference point and the maximum and minimum dose positions
(6) Descriptions and diagrams of the placement of dosimeters and other test samples
(7) Specified minimum dose and minimum and maximum tolerances and reference to the dosimeter system used routinely
(8) Requirements for routine quality control tests and periodic audits related to sterilization
(9) Written criteria for sterile product acceptance, reprocessing, rejection, and release for distribution, including instructions for selection, handling, and testing of samples

Failure to meet the physical specifications should result in quarantine of the sterilization load and in an investigation. The investigation should be documented. If the delivered dose is below the validated dose, the sterilization load should not be released; product should be either resterilized or scrapped. Because radiation effects on materials are cumulative, any decision to resterilize must be based on acceptable product aging test data after multiple sterilizations. Process interruptions or delays should be evaluated to determine the effect on the microbiological quality of the product and on the dosimetry systems.

ADOPTING A DEVICE INTO A VALIDATED STERILIZATION SYSTEM

When a new or altered device is added to the product line, an evaluation must be conducted to ensure the device's compatibility with the sterilization process and to ascertain the challenge it presents to the current validated dose. The adopted device and its packaging must be analyzed for compatibility with the dose range. In addition, it must be determined if the adopted device is less difficult to sterilize than the master challenge device used to validate the sterilization cycle.

A person knowledgeable and experienced in the factors affecting radiation sterilization and microbial lethality must perform the evaluation. A checklist should be developed that lists all the device construction and package and load configuration issues that affect sterilizability. The checklist should include the following items:

(1) Primary packaging
(2) Packaging—corrugated, polyliner, number of boxes per case, tote configuration, and product density
(3) Device construction
(4) Routine dose conditions—validated dose range, dose map similarities
(5) Bioburden—levels, higher or lower, resistance, ID
(6) Manufacturing environment—controlled

Once the evaluation is complete and if the adopted device is clearly judged to be easier-to-sterilize than the master challenge device, it can be adopted into the validated sterilization process on the basis of the documented review. If, however, a question is raised or it appears to be more difficult to sterilize than the master challenge device, a confirmation of bioburden numbers and resistance should be run. Enumerate and identify the bioburden organisms and compare data to a similar study performed on the master challenge product. Perform a fractional dose experiment with twenty each of the new product and twenty each of the master product. After dosing, sterility test both products to determine the relative resistance. If more growth appears in the new product sterility containers, then it is judged to be more difficult to sterilize. A new dose experiment must be performed using the new product as the family representative.

DOSE AUDIT FAILURE

The dose audit for both Methods 1 and 2 requires that 100 product units be irradiated at the original 10^{-2} dose and then tested for sterility. If three or more positives occur, the result is considered a dose audit failure and certain actions must be taken. Depending on the number of positives, the action required is either a retest or the re-establishment of the sterilization dose. In either case, augmentation of the original sterilization dose is required while the retest or reestablishment of the sterilization is occurring.

In addition to augmenting the sterilization dose, two other actions should occur:

(1) An investigation to determine the cause of the audit failure
(2) Analysis of the impact of the audit failure on other batches sterilized prior to augmentation of the dose

Three possible outcomes of an investigation into the cause of the audit failure are:

(1) A change in the manufacturing process, environment or components
(2) An error in the test procedure of dose delivery
(3) The cause cannot be determined

When the cause of the failure is attributed to a change in the manufacturing process, environment or components, it should be possible to determine the time frame in which the change occurred and therefore the batches affected. A revised sterility assurance level should be estimated for batches already released and a decision made on the risk associated with their continued use. This can be done by determining the log reduction actually achieved using the Stumbo-Cockran-Murphy equation below, the highest bioburden value obtained and the result of the sterility test. If the product requires a SAL = 10^{-6}, then a log reduction of ≥ 12 should be attained.

$$D = \frac{U}{\log No - \log Nu}$$

where

U = verification dose
No = initial bioburden population
Nu = $2.303 \log n/r$
n = total number of tests
r = number of sterility tests

$$\log \text{ reduction} = \log No - \log Nu$$

Another approach could be a literature review and use of the highest D-value cited. Some examples of literature-reported values compiled from multiple sources are listed in Table 21. The highest resistance reported for the Method 1 population by Whitby is 4.2 kGy; using a similar technique, a D-value of 4.0 kGy was determined in Japan using isolates from medical devices.

If the cause of the audit failure is attributed to an error in the test method, it is not a true dose audit failure and the test can be repeated. Moreover, there is no impact on the sterility assurance of already released batches. The cause of the test failure must be corrected prior to the retest. Several examples of problems that could result in a test method failure are:

- Samples are contaminated during preparation for test.
- Packaging could be compromised during shipment.
- Lab contamination could occur during preparation of the sterility suite.
- Samples are not decontaminated properly.
- Bioburden was underestimated.

Sometimes the cause of the audit failure cannot be determined. In situations such as this it is impossible to assess the impact on the sterility assurance level of previously sterilized batches. Augmentation of the dose should begin with the next batch and no action taken with the already released batches.

TABLE 21. Sensitivity of Microorganisms to Radiation.

Group	Organism	D-Value (kGy)
Sensitive	Vegetative bacteria	0.1–1.6
	• *Escherichia coli*	0.3–0.6
	• *Streptococci* species	1.0–2.2
	• *Pseudomonas* species	0.3
	• *Staphylococci* species	0.8–1.6
	• *Flavobacterium* species	0.3
Moderately Resistant	Molds and Yeasts	0.5–3.8
	• *Saccharomyces*	0.5
	• *Aspergillus niger*	0.5
	• *Penicillium*	2.0
	• *Cryptococcus*	1.4–3.1
	Streptococcus faecium	1.2–3.8
Resistant	*Micrococci radiodurans*	2.0–8.8
	Anaerobic spore formers	1.2–3.7
	• *Clostridium botulinum*	1.2–3.7
	• *C. sporogenes*	1.6–2.2
	Aerobic spore formers	0.6–3.0
	• *Bacillus subtilis* (1289)	2.2
	• *B. pumilus*	1.7–3.0
	• *B. stearothermophilus*	2.2

FREQUENCY OF STERILIZATION DOSE AUDITS

A reduction in the frequency of sterilization dose audits is possible when:

(1) Successful, consecutive sterilization dose audits (i.e., no dose augmentations) have been carried out, at intervals of no more than three months, over a period of twelve months.

(2) Data are available that demonstrate stability of bioburden over at least a period of twelve months. These include:
   • a minimum of quarterly bioburden determinations
   • characterization of bioburden (for example, use of selective media, Gram stain of isolates, an examination of cellular morphology, etc.)

(3) The manufacture of the product in relation to bioburden is controlled and the effectiveness of this control is demonstrated through implementation of elements of a quality system as defined in ISO 13485 or 13488.

If the above criteria are met and documented, the initial reduction in frequency from a three month interval to a six month interval is appropriate. A further reduction to a twelve month interval can be considered if the above criteria are demonstrated for a 24-month period. Reduction in frequency should occur in a step fashion as continued acceptable dose audits are performed over time with the maximum interval never exceeding twelve months. If any dose audit fails during the frequency reduction period, the sterilization dose should be augmented or re-established and the frequency of sterilization dose audits must revert to a minimum of three months.

Contract Radiation Sterilization Facilities in the United States (Partial Listing)

Company	City	State	Type
Beta Beam Inc.	Lima	OH	Electron Beam
COBE Laboratories	Lakewood	CO	Gamma
E-Beam Services	Cranbury	NJ	Electron Beam
MMC Medical Manufacturing Corp.	Erie	PA	Gamma
Gammamed Inc.	Columbus	MS	Gamma
IRT Corporation	San Diego	CA	Electron Beam
Isomedix/Steris	Groveport	OH	Gamma
Isomedix/Steris	Libertyville	IL	Gamma/Electron Beam
Isomedix/Steris	El Paso	TX	Gamma/EtO
Isomedix/Steris	Sandy	UT	Gamma
Isomedix/Steris	Whippany	NY	Gamma
Isomedix/Steris	Chester	NY	Gamma/EtO
Isomedix/Steris	Northborough	MA	Gamma/EtO
Isomedix/Steris	Morton Grove	IL	Gamma
Isomedix/Steris	Spartanburg	SC	Gamma/EtO
Medical Sterilization Inc.	Syosset	NY	Electron Beam
NUTEK Corp.	Palo Alto	CA	Electron Beam
NUTEK Corp.	Salt Lake City	UT	Electron Beam
Neutron Products Inc.	Dickerson	MD	Electron Beam
Radiation Technology Inc.	Haw River	NC	Gamma
Radiation Technology Inc.	Roakaway	NJ	Gamma
IBA/SteriGenics International	Schaumburg, Gurnee	IL	Gamma
IBA/SteriGenics International	Charlotte, Haw River	NC	Gamma
IBA/SteriGenics International	Fort Worth	TX	Gamma
IBA/SteriGenics International	Hayward, Corona	CA	Gamma
IBA/SteriGenics International	Westerville	OH	Gamma
IBA/SteriGenics International	San Diego	CA	Electron Beam
IBA/SteriGenics International	West Memphis	AR	Gamma
IBA/SteriGenics International	Somerset	NJ	Gamma
Titan Scan Systems	Denver	CO	Electron Beam

Method 1 Dose Verification

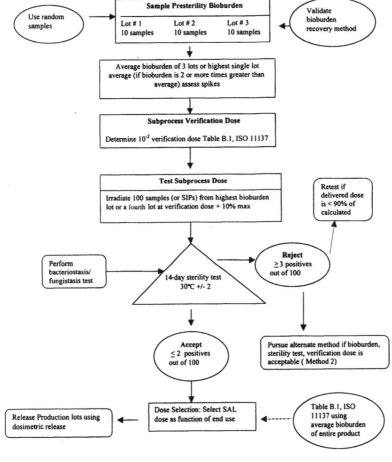

Use random samples

Sample Presterility Bioburden

| Lot # 1 | Lot # 2 | Lot # 3 |
| 10 samples | 10 samples | 10 samples |

Validate bioburden recovery method

Average bioburden of 3 lots or highest single lot average (if bioburden is 2 or more times greater than average) assess spikes

Subprocess Verification Dose

Determine 10^{-2} verification dose Table B.1, ISO 11137

Test Subprocess Dose

Irradiate 100 samples (or SIPs) from highest bioburden lot or a fourth lot at verification dose + 10% max

Retest if delivered dose is < 90% of calculated

Perform bacteriostasis/ fungistasis test

14-day sterility test 30°C +/- 2

Reject ≥ 3 positives out of 100

Accept ≤ 2 positives out of 100

Pursue alternate method if bioburden, sterility test, verification dose is acceptable (Method 2)

Release Production lots using dosimetric release

Dose Selection: Select SAL dose as function of end use

Table B.1, ISO 11137 using average bioburden of entire product

109

Method 1 Quarterly Dose Audit

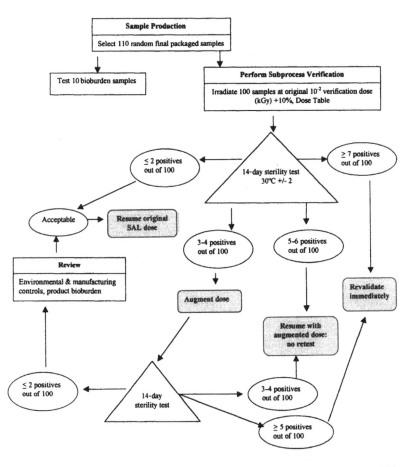

Sample Production
Select 110 random final packaged samples

Test 10 bioburden samples

Perform Subprocess Verification
Irradiate 100 samples at original 10^{-2} verification dose
(kGy) +10%, Dose Table

≤ 2 positives out of 100

≥ 7 positives out of 100

14-day sterility test
30°C +/- 2

Acceptable

Resume original SAL dose

3-4 positives out of 100

5-6 positives out of 100

Review
Environmental & manufacturing controls, product bioburden

Augment dose

Revalidate immediately

Resume with augmented dose: no retest

≤ 2 positives out of 100

14-day sterility test

3-4 positives out of 100

≥ 5 positives out of 100

Worked Example for Method 1

Term	Value	Comment
Stage 1, SIP < 1		
SAL	10^{-6}	Product for sale in EU or product required SAL 10^{-6}
SIP	0.05	Product too large so a 1/20 portion was selected
Stage 2		
SIP bioburden	59	Results of 50, 62, 65 from three batches. None of the individual SIP results was 2× the average.
Average bioburden	1180	The bioburden for product units was calculated:
		50/0.05 = 1000
		62/0.05 = 1240
		65/0.05 = 1300
		None of the individual batch results was 2× the average, therefore 1180 will be used to select the verification dose.
Stage 3		
Verification dose	7.3 kGy	Verification dose for SIP of 59 is found in Table B.1. Since 59 are not found, the next larger bioburden of 59.2 is used.
Stage 4		
Sterility results	2+ at 6.8 kGy	The actual dose was within the specified range (i.e., less than 8.0 kGy) and the sterility test results were acceptable (i.e., < 2+).
Stage 5		
Sterilization dose for 10^{-6} SAL	25.3 kGy	Sterilization dose for 1180 from Table B.1. Since 1180 is not found, the next larger bioburden of 1182 is used.

113

Method 2A Dose Validation

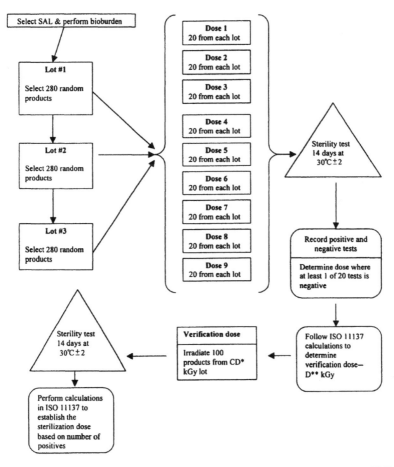

Worked Example for Single Product Batch (SIP < 1)

Term	Value	Comment

Stage 1
  SAL
  SIP
	10^{-6}
	0.05
		The product required a 10^{-6} SAL.
		The product was too large to sterility test, so a 1/20 portion was selected.

Stage 2
  Average SIP bioburden
 	
  Average total bioburden
	59
	
	1180
		The bioburden data for 10 SIPs was 50, 65, 72, 35, 60, 55, 48, 69, 75 and 61 for an average of 59.
		Average for the entire device = 59/0.05 = 1180.

Stage 3 Verification dose	7.3 kGy	The verification dose is found in Table 2. Since 59 is not there, the next higher value (59.2) is used.
Stage 4 Test of sterility	2+ at 6.8 kGy	The dose and sterility test results were within acceptable ranges.

Stage 5
  Sterilization dose for 10^{-6}
  SAL
	25.3 kGy	Dose determined from Table 2.

Worked Example of VD_{max} 25 kGy Substantiation (SIP < 1)

Term	Value	Comment
Stage 1		
SAL	10^{-6}	This method only substantiates a 10^{-6} SAL at 25 kGy.
SIP	0.5	The product was too large to sterility test, so a 1/2 portion was used.
Stage 2		
SIP bioburden	59	SIP bioburden results of 50, 62, and 65 were observed.
Average bioburden	118	Bioburden average of 59. SIP 0.5 = 118.
Stage 3		
Verification dose	8.1 kGy	Average bioburden and Table 2. 118 is not listed so the next higher bioburden of 120 was used. Apply equation: SIP verification dose = 9.0 + (log 0.05 * 2.91) = 8.1.
Stage 4		
Sterility test	0+ at 7.9 kGy	The verification dose was within the specified range.
Stage 5		
Sterilization dose	25 kGy	The sterility test was acceptable.

119

Worked Example for Dose Augmentation for Device Qualified Using Method 1 (adapted from Herring)

$SAL = 10^{-6}$
$SIP = 1$
Product bioburden = Average 45 CFU/device
Method 1 verification dose = 7.0 kGy
Audit bioburden = Average 47 CFU/device
Audit dose range = 6.4 – 6.8 kGy
Audit results = 6+/100

Dose Augmentation Calculation

Estimate of resistance = <10 audit positives
FNP = max. audit dose + 2.0 kGy
$FNP = 6.8 + 2.0 = 8.8$ kGy
$FFP = 1$ (assumed)
$FNP - FFP < 10$
DS kGy = $2 + 0.2(FNP - FFP)$ kGy
DS kGy $= 2 + 0.2(8.8 - 1) = 3.6$ kGy (estimate or resistance – D-value)

Adjust 10^{-2} SAL Dose

D^{**} kGy = DD^* kGy + [log (CD^*)] (DS) kGy
D^{**} kGy $= 6.8 + [\log 6 (3.6)] = 9.6$ kGy (dose to achieve 10^{-2} SAL)

Calculate Augmented Sterilization Dose

ASD kGy = D^{**} kGy + [$-$log SAL $-$ log SIP $-$ 2] DS kGy
ASD kGy $= 9.6 + [-\log 10^{-6} - \log 1 - 2] 3.6 = 24.0$ kGy

Dose Validation Protocol

PROTOCOL

Validation of Radiation
(E-Beam or Gamma) Sterilization
for
Company (Name), Inc.

Company (name), Inc.	Prepared by: *Booth Scientific, Inc.*
Address	968 Shoreline Road
City, State, Zip Code	Barrington, IL 60010
Phone:	Phone: 847-304-5685
Study Director:	Contract # : _____

Index

1.0 PURPOSE
2.0 SCOPE
3.0 RESPONSIBILITIES
4.0 MATERIALS AND EQUIPMENT
5.0 PROCEDURE
6.0 ACCEPTANCE CRITERIA
7.0 APPROVALS
8.0 REFERENCES

Inserts

- Exhibit 1—Product description
- Exhibit 2—Dose Map

1.0 Purpose

The purpose of this protocol is to define the requirements and the acceptance criteria for the validation of irradiation (E-beam or gamma) at the Contract Sterilizer (name) facility for Company's (name) product line. This validation will ensure a 10^{-6} sterility assurance level (SAL).

2.0 Scope

2.1 This protocol applies to Company (name)'s product line as defined in Exhibit 1. The procedure used for this qualification is Method 1 outlined in ISO 11137 (or other applicable method) standard and shall serve to qualify products for sale.

2.2 This protocol will not include the Installation Qualification and dosimetry qualification studies performed by Contract Sterilizer (name). Contract Sterilizer (name) shall ensure that all studies have been acceptably performed, and all documentation pertaining to these studies is available at Contract Sterilizer (name) for review.

2.3 This protocol shall incorporate any other applicable studies, including the initial bioburden and verification dose experiments.

2.4 An environmental monitoring program has been established, and regular monitoring for viable air and surface particulate is ongoing. A trend analysis has been performed and shows control of the environment.

3.0 Responsibilities

3.1 It is the responsibility of Company (name) to provide Contract Sterilizer (name) with an approved protocol outlining the performance qualification testing. Company (name) shall ensure that the product is manufactured in a properly controlled environment. Company (name) shall provide the product loads and samples to Contract Sterilizer (name) in a timely manner. Company (name) shall confirm product efficacy subsequent to processing and provide sterile product to Company (name) for distribution.

3.2 It is the responsibility of Contract Sterilizer (name) to provide

Company (name) with all pertinent data, records, charts, SOPs, maintenance, and dosimeter calibration records (if asked) within 5 days of completion of each batch process run. Any deviations from protocol or specification shall be communicated to the study director immediately.

3.3 It is the responsibility of the Consultant to provide Company (name) with an acceptable protocol, meeting all requirements of the regulatory agencies, and to provide guidance or hands-on assistance in the execution of the protocol according to contract. Any changes to the approved protocol shall be handled with an addendum. A final report shall be written summarizing all data. Separate protocols shall be written covering biocompatibility and shelf life studies.

4.0 Materials and Equipment

4.1 Company (name) product line description (Exhibit 1)

4.2 Thirty (30) each bioburden product samples, 10 each from three (3) different batches

4.3 100 each finished product samples for dose verifications at Contract Sterilizer (name) radiation facilities (if using Method 1, alternate product samples if using other methods)

4.4 220 each product samples for dosing at a maximum dose (use maximum dose expected during routine processing or two times sterilized product) for shelf life (accelerated aging, if used), functionality, and biocompatibility testing

4.5 Qualified testing laboratory used for bioburden and product sterility testing: name

5.0 Procedure

5.1 Determination of Bioburden

5.1.1 Procure ten (10) each product samples randomly from three (3) different batches. These shall be representative of the routine production processes.

5.1.2 Send to test lab for bioburden evaluation (ask for enumeration of aerobes, fungus, and spores.)

5.1.2.1 At the test lab, perform the bioburden determinations using a standard method as outlined in ISO 11737-1 by extracting each device individually and filtering the extract through a sterile bacterial retentive filter.

5.1.2.2 A validation of bioburden recovery should be performed. (An additional five nonsterile samples are required.)

5.1.3 Determine the average bioburden per device for each lot, as well as the overall batch average bioburden (apply the recovery factor prior to calculating the average).

5.1.3.1 Calculate the overall average bioburden. If a spike (a single value at least 2 × the overall average) occurs, the spike value may be used rather than the average for the dose selection.

5.2 Determine the Verification Dose Using Method 1 (or alternate method)

5.2.1 Review the bioburden results. If any single batch average is 2 × greater than the overall bioburden average, use it to determine the verification dose. If not, use the overall average. Go to Table B.1 of the standard for the verification dose.

5.2.2 Randomly select 100 packaged devices from a single batch of products. These can be selected from any of the batches used for bioburden or from a fourth batch recently manufactured in a similar manner.

5.2.3 Send the samples to Contract Sterilizer (name) for the verification dose experiment.

5.2.4 After dosing, Contract Sterilizer (name) shall send the processed samples to lab for sterility testing. The certificate of irradiation shall be mailed to Company Study Director.

5.2.5 The test lab shall sterility test the samples in Soybean Casein

Digest Broth and incubate at $30° \pm 2°C$ for 14 days to determine the number of samples with surviving organisms. Bacteriostasis/ fungistasis testing must be performed on this product.

5.3 Evaluation of the sterility test results

5.3.1 The verification dose is acceptable if two (2) or less samples show growth.

5.3.2 If more than two (2) samples show growth, the verification test is rejected. An investigation shall be performed to evaluate if the failure could be due to incorrect handling of product, incorrect performance of the test, or incorrect dosing.

5.3.2.1 If so determined, the verification dose experiment can be repeated.

5.4 Sterilizing Dose Designation

5.4.1 If the verification dose is found acceptable, then a sterilization dose is determined from Table B.1, and the product sterilization is validated.

5.4.1.1 All subsequent batches shall be dosed at the sterilizing dose as the minimum specification.

5.5 Product and Packaging Qualification

5.5.1 The effect of radiation on the product and packaging shall be evaluated. The testing program shall include stability of materials (obtain information from suppliers of raw materials), shelf life aging studies (under separate protocol) to show no detrimental effects on product function over time, evaluation of product function at maximum doses, biocompatibility, and any other pertinent tests. A package integrity evaluation (under separate protocol) should evaluate seal strength and assure that the intact package has not been compromised.

5.5.2 One (1) case containing twelve boxes of 100 devices shall be the unit package for irradiation. Two (2) each cases shall be placed in each carrier for presentation to the radiation source (or use a statistically acceptable number depending on batch size).

5.5.3 A dose map has been performed to indicate the D_{min} and D_{max} ratio depending on the minimum dose specified (see Exhibit 2).

5.5.4 Prepare 220 each product samples and place in final packaging. Send the samples to Contract Sterilizer (name) and dose at _____ kGy (maximum dose expected during routine processing).

5.5.4.1 Evaluate thirty samples for product functionality according to Company (name) standard methods.

5.5.4.2 Send sixty samples to testing lab for package and shipping evaluation. The effect of shipping and handling on the package shall be evaluated using a physical test method (select one outlined in ASTM method), and the product shall be tested for functionality.

5.5.4.3 Send nine samples to lab for three (3) biocompatibility tests (if they have not been performed previously on radiated product) determined to be appropriate for devices of limited contact, external communicating: cytotoxicity—2 samples (MEM elution), irritation—2 samples, and sensitization—5 samples.

5.5.4.4 Evaluate the latent effects of radiation on 120 samples by performing a real-time aging study using thirty samples at each of four time frames (select the maximum time expected and three lower ones). Evaluate the package to assure that the sterile barrier is intact. Test procedures and results shall be performed under a separate protocol. Accelerated aging studies may be performed, if required.

5.6 Dose Audits

5.6.1 Each quarter after the initial validation is successfully completed, a dose audit shall be performed to determine the continued validity of the initial dose.

5.6.2 Pull 110 product units from a single batch.

5.6.2.1 Using the same bioburden methods as before, determine the bioburden on ten (10) samples.

5.6.2.2 Irradiate the remaining 100 units at the verification dose found in the initial validation. The actual dose not vary by +10%, but cannot be less than 90%.

5.6.2.3 Sterility test the products as in 5.3.5.

5.6.3 If fewer than 2 positives result, no action is needed; the dose is acceptable.

5.6.4 If 3–4 positives result, the sterilization dose shall be augmented following the guidance in Section B.3.5.4 of the standard. Thereafter, a retest at the original verification dose may be performed to determine if augmentation of the dose should continue. Follow section B.3.5.3.

6.0 Acceptance Criteria

6.1 An environmental monitoring program to verify consistency in the manufacturing process and bioburden levels is verified; the audit demonstrates that no extraordinary change from established specifications has occurred.

6.2 The original delivered dose is not greater than 10% and not less than 90% of the specified verification dose.

6.3 Sterility results meet specifications in section 5.3. B/F tests are acceptable.

6.4 Product and package function evaluations after delivery of the sterilizing dose are acceptable. Shelf life and biocompatibility studies are in progress.

7.0 Approvals

Protocol prepared by: _____ Date _____
                    (Consultant)
Approved by:_____ Date _____
          (Company Representative)
Approved by: _____ Date _____
          (Company Representative)
Accepted by: _____ Date _____
          (Sterilization Facility Manager)

8.0 References

AAMI TIR 17: *Radiation Sterilization—Material Qualification,* AAMI, Arlington, VA 1998.

ANSI/AAMI/ISO 11137-1995: *Sterilization of health care products—Requirements for validation and routine control—Radiation sterilization,* AAMI, Arlington, VA, 1995.

ANSI/AAMI/ISO 11737-1: 1995: *Sterilization of medical devices—Microbiological methods—Part 1: Estimation of population of microorganisms on products,* AAMI, Arlington, VA, 1995.

FDA Quality System Regulation, Fed. Reg., October 6, 1996.

ANSI/AAMI/ISO 11737-2: *Sterilization of medical devices—Microbiological methods—Part 2: Tests for sterility performed in the validation of sterilization processes,* AAMI, Arlington, VA, 1998.

EXHIBIT 1. Company (Name), Inc.'s Product Line (Include a Diagram or Drawing of the Finished Device).

EXHIBIT 2. Contract Sterilizer (Name) Dose Map of Company (Name) Product.

Accelerated Aging Protocol

PROTOCOL

Accelerated Aging Study
for
Irradiated Product

1.0 Purpose

1.1. To outline the procedure for evaluating the expiration dating of company's (name) product using an accelerated aging methodology.

2.0 Scope

2.1 Validation of the expiration date shall be achieved by accelerated aging of samples from three separate batches of sterilized products to the desired expiration date of _____ years (state desired time frame). Product and package integrity and functionality testing shall be performed after aging and compared to non-aged product to determine an acceptable product expiry date. In conjunction with accelerated aging studies, an evaluation shall be performed on products that have been stored for _____ years (state desired time frame) at ambient conditions.

2.2 The methods used to simulate aging involve elevated temperatures using a thermodynamic temperature coefficient. A rule that was first stated by Von't Hoff states that, "a rise in temperature of 10°C will double the rate of a chemical reaction." This rule is usually expressed as a Q_{10} value, i.e., the ratio of the rate of a reaction at two temperatures 10°C apart. If the rate of the reaction is doubled, then $Q_{10} = 2$. This is the most common approach used in the medical device industry for conducting package integrity studies.

2.2.1 The elevated temperature condition used for the accelerated aging of medical device packages is 55°C (131°F). If $Q_{10} = 2$ and the accelerated aging conditions are 55°C, or 35°C over an ambient temperature of 20°C, then the aging factor is $2^{3.5}$ or 11.3 times. Fifty-two weeks divided by 11.3 = 4.6 weeks. Therefore, 4.6 weeks at 55°C is equivalent to one year at ambient temperatures (other temperatures and times can be used).

2.2.2 The packages containing the radiated products are rotated through high and low humidity conditions at 55°C and are briefly stored at freezing temperatures. The freezing and humidity are included as additional stresses in order to simulate worst-case conditions.

2.2.3 The standard one year equivalency accelerated aging cycle will be repeated a total of _____ times to simulate _____ years (stipulate your time frame) of room temperature equivalency.

2.3 If package validation studies are included, three batches of products will be used per product type. Three separate operators will seal every batch of product to be utilized in the study on three separate days. This will take into account variability of the machine operation on different days and by different operators.

2.4 Accelerated aging testing will be performed at lab (name). The laboratory will be responsible for test procedures, test materials and equipment qualification, and test result documentation.

2.5 Functionality testing will be performed at company (name) using standard procedures. (List procedures to be followed.)

3.0 Equipment/Supplies/Forms

3.1 A minimum of _____ products (select a statistically acceptable number based on batch size. A minimum of thirty for each test is recommended.)

3.2 Environmental Chamber at 55°C ± 2°C and 75 ± 5% R.H. (or other desired temperature and relative humidity)

3.3 Freezer at −20°C–10°C

3.4 Environmental Chamber at 55°C ± 2°C and < 20% R.H.

3.5 Equipment and supplies as specified for packaging and product testing

4.0 Procedure

4.1 Ambient Conditions Aging

4.1.1 A minimum of thirty products (or a selected master product typical of all products) radiation sterilized at the maximum dose from each of three different batches shall be stored at room temperature (20–25°C) for _____ years (stipulate desired time frame).

4.1.2 Perform product and package functionality testing at each selected time frame as outlined in section 4.3.

4.2 Accelerated Aging

4.2.1 A minimum of thirty products for each year of predicted shelf life irradiated at the maximum dose shall be subjected to an accelerated aging procedure. (For a five-year study, start with a minimum of 150 product samples.)

4.2.1.1 Check packages prior to sending product to test lab for any visible signs of damage. Only intact samples will be utilized for testing.

4.2.2 Select a minimum of thirty non-sterile products from a single lot and subject them to the same aging procedure.

4.2.3 Place all samples in a 55°C ± 2°C and 75 ± 5% R.H. environmental chamber. Record the date, times, and chamber information.

4.2.4 Remove samples after 2.3 weeks (16 to 18 days) and record the date and time of removal of the samples from the chamber.

4.2.5 Place the test samples in a −15°C ± 5°C freezer and record the date, time, and chamber information.

4.2.6 After 24 hours, remove the samples and record the date and time of removal of the samples from the freezer.

4.2.7 Again place the samples in a 55°C ± 2°C and < 20% R.H. environmental chamber and record as before.

4.2.8 Remove all samples after another 2.3 weeks (16 to 18 days).

4.2.9 Repeat the above accelerated aging cycle (sections 6.2.3 through 6.2.8) _____ times for each year at ambient room temperature.

4.2.9.1 Check all samples for any signs of visible damage at the conclusion of each yearly time point. Notify Company (name) immediately if any packaging is compromised.

4.3 Test Sample Disposition and Procedure

4.3.1 Following _____ years of "real time" aging and after the _____ year equivalency accelerated aging cycle, all samples from each of three batches of each type of product shall be submitted for packaging and functionality testing. (Recommend testing after each year.)

4.3.1.1 Test a minimum of thirty samples from each of the three product batches per product type for package functionality using dye penetration (or other physical test method outlined in ISO 11607) testing and for peel strength.

4.3.1.2 After completion of package testing, evaluate product functionality using company procedures.

4.3.2 Also test the non-sterile product to serve as the control to assess the effects of the irradiation process.

5.0 Acceptance Criteria

5.1 An expiration date of _____ years can be assigned to company's (name) products if all samples (or an acceptable number based on selected AQL level) from each of three batches for each type of product pass the two physical package integrity tests as well as the functionality tests following _____ years of accelerated aging.

5.2 The _____ year expiration date must be further confirmed by passing test results on products which have been stored at ambient conditions when such products become available.

6.0 Approvals

Prepared by: _____ _____
                       Consultant (If Used)   Date

Approved by: _____ _____
                       Quality Assurance Manager, Company   Date

7.0 References

Reich, R. R., Sharpe, D. C., and Anderson, H. D., "Accelerated Aging of Packaging Used in Expiration Date Verification," *Medical Device & Diagnostic Industry,* March 1988, p. 35.

American Society for Testing and Materials, F1980-99el *Standard Guide for Accelerated Aging of Sterile Medical Packages,* ASTM, West Conshohocken, PA, 2000.

Association for the Advancement of Medical Instrumentation, Technical Information Report Number 17, *Radiation sterilization—Material qualification.*

Association for the Advancement of Medical Instrumentation, *Packaging for terminally sterilized medical devices,* ANSI/AAMI/ISO 11607-1997.

Radiation Dose (kGy) Required to Achieve Given SAL (Adapted from May 2000 Draft Revision of ISO 11137 Annex B)

Bioburden	10^{-2}	10^{-3}	10^{-4}	10^{-5}	10^{-6}
1.0	3.0	5.2	8.0	11.0	14.2
1.1	3.3	5.7	8.5	11.5	14.8
2.0	3.6	6.0	8.8	11.9	15.2
2.5	3.8	6.3	9.1	12.2	15.6
3.0	4.0	6.5	9.4	12.5	15.8
3.5	4.1	6.7	9.6	12.7	16.1
4.0	4.3	6.8	9.7	12.9	16.2
4.5	4.4	7.0	9.9	13.1	16.4
5.0	4.5	7.1	10.0	13.2	16.6
5.5	4.6	7.2	10.2	13.4	16.7
6.0	4.7	7.3	10.3	13.5	16.9
6.5	4.8	7.4	10.4	13.6	17.1
7.0	4.8	7.5	10.5	13.8	17.2
7.5	4.9	7.7	10.7	13.9	17.3
8.0	5.0	7.7	10.7	13.9	17.4
8.5	5.1	7.8	10.8	14.0	17.4
9.0	5.1	7.8	10.8	14.1	17.5
9.5	5.2	7.9	10.9	14.1	17.6
10	5.2	8.0	11.0	14.2	17.8
11	5.3	8.1	11.1	14.5	17.9
12	5.4	8.2	11.2	14.5	17.9
13	5.5	8.3	11.3	14.6	18.0
14	5.6	8.4	11.4	14.7	18.1
15	5.7	8.5	11.5	14.8	18.2
16	5.8	8.5	11.6	14.9	18.3
17	5.8	8.6	11.7	15.0	18.5
18	5.9	8.7	11.8	15.1	18.5
19	5.9	8.8	11.9	15.1	18.6
20	6.0	8.8	11.9	15.2	18.7

(continued)

139

Bioburden	10^{-2}	10^{-3}	10^{-4}	10^{-5}	10^{-6}
22	6.1	9.0	12.1	15.4	19.0
24	6.2	9.1	12.2	15.5	19.0
26	6.3	9.2	12.3	15.6	19.2
28	6.4	9.3	12.4	15.7	19.2
30	6.5	9.4	12.5	15.8	19.4
32	6.6	9.4	12.6	15.9	19.5
34	6.6	9.5	12.7	16.0	19.5
36	6.7	9.6	12.8	16.1	19.6
38	6.8	9.7	12.8	16.2	19.8
40	6.8	9.7	12.9	16.2	19.8
42	6.9	9.8	13.0	16.3	19.8
44	6.9	9.9	13.0	16.4	19.9
46	7.0	9.9	13.1	16.5	20.0
48	7.0	10.0	13.2	16.5	20.0
50	7.1	10.0	13.2	16.6	20.1
55	7.2	10.2	13.4	16.7	20.3
60	7.3	10.3	13.5	16.9	20.4
65	7.4	10.4	13.6	17.0	20.5
70	7.5	10.5	13.7	17.1	20.6
75	7.6	10.6	13.8	17.2	20.7
80	7.7	10.7	13.9	17.3	20.8
85	7.7	10.8	14.0	17.3	20.8
90	7.8	10.8	14.1	17.5	21.0
95	7.9	10.9	14.1	17.5	21.1
100	8.0	11.0	14.2	17.6	21.2
110	8.1	11.1	14.3	17.8	21.3
120	8.2	11.2	14.5	17.8	21.3
130	8.3	11.3	14.6	18.0	21.6
140	8.4	11.4	14.7	18.1	21.7
150	8.5	11.5	14.8	18.2	21.8
160	8.5	11.6	14.9	18.3	21.9
170	8.6	11.7	15.0	18.4	22.0
180	8.7	11.8	15.1	18.5	22.1
190	8.8	11.9	15.1	18.6	22.2
200	8.8	11.9	15.2	18.7	22.3
220	9.0	12.1	15.4	18.8	22.4
240	9.1	12.2	15.5	19.0	22.6
260	9.2	12.3	15.6	19.1	22.7
280	9.3	12.4	15.7	19.2	22.8
300	9.4	12.5	15.8	19.3	22.9
325	9.5	12.6	15.9	19.4	23.1
350	9.6	12.7	16.0	19.5	23.2
375	9.7	12.8	16.2	19.7	23.3
400	9.7	12.9	16.2	19.8	23.4
425	9.8	13.0	16.3	19.8	23.5
450	9.9	13.1	16.4	19.9	23.6
475	10.0	13.1	16.5	20.0	23.7
500	10.0	13.2	16.6	20.1	23.7

Bioburden	10^{-2}	10^{-3}	10^{-4}	10^{-5}	10^{-6}
525	10.1	13.3	16.7	20.2	23.8
550	10.2	13.4	16.7	20.3	23.9
575	10.2	13.4	16.8	20.3	24.0
600	10.3	13.5	16.9	20.4	24.0
650	10.4	13.6	17.0	20.5	24.2
700	10.5	13.7	17.1	20.6	24.3
750	10.6	13.8	17.2	20.7	24.4
800	10.7	13.9	17.3	20.8	24.5
850	10.8	14.0	17.4	20.9	24.6
900	10.8	14.1	17.5	21.0	24.7
950	10.9	14.1	17.5	21.1	24.8
1000	11.0	14.2	17.6	21.2	24.9
1050	11.0	14.3	17.7	21.3	24.9
1100	11.1	14.4	17.8	21.3	25.0
1150	11.2	14.4	17.8	21.4	25.1
1200	11.2	14.5	17.9	21.5	25.2
1250	11.3	14.5	18.0	21.5	25.2
1300	11.3	14.6	18.0	21.6	25.3
1350	11.4	14.6	18.1	21.7	25.3
1400	11.4	14.7	18.1	21.7	25.4
1450	11.5	14.8	18.2	21.8	25.5
1500	11.5	14.8	18.2	21.8	25.5
1600	11.6	14.9	18.3	21.9	25.6
1700	11.7	15.0	18.4	22.0	25.7
1800	11.8	15.1	18.5	22.1	25.8
1900	11.9	15.1	18.6	22.2	25.9
2000	11.9	15.2	18.7	22.3	26.0
2100	12.0	15.3	18.8	22.4	26.1
2200	12.1	15.4	18.8	22.4	26.1
2300	12.1	15.4	18.9	22.5	26.2
2400	12.2	15.5	19.0	22.6	26.3
2500	12.2	15.6	19.0	22.6	26.4
2600	12.3	15.6	19.1	22.7	26.4
2700	12.3	15.7	19.1	22.8	26.5
2800	12.4	15.7	19.2	22.8	26.5
2900	12.4	15.8	19.3	22.9	26.6
3000	12.5	15.8	19.3	22.9	26.6
3400	12.7	16.0	19.5	23.0	26.8
3600	12.8	16.1	19.6	23.2	26.9
3800	12.8	16.2	19.7	23.3	27.0
4000	12.9	16.3	19.8	23.4	27.1
4200	13.0	16.3	19.8	23.5	27.2
4400	13.0	16.4	19.9	23.5	27.3
4600	13.1	16.5	20.0	23.6	27.3
4800	13.2	16.5	20.0	23.7	27.4
5000	13.2	16.6	20.1	23.7	27.5
5300	13.3	16.7	20.2	23.8	27.6
5600	13.4	16.8	20.3	23.9	27.7

(continued)

Bioburden	10^{-2}	10^{-3}	10^{-4}	10^{-5}	10^{-6}
5900	13.5	16.8	20.4	24.0	27.8
6500	13.6	17.0	20.5	24.2	27.9
6800	13.7	17.0	20.6	24.2	28.0
7100	13.7	17.1	20.7	24.3	28.1
7400	13.8	17.2	20.7	24.4	28.1
7700	13.8	17.2	20.8	24.4	28.2
8000	13.9	17.3	20.8	24.5	28.3
8500	14.0	17.4	20.9	24.6	28.4
9000	14.1	17.5	21.0	24.7	28.5
10000	14.2	17.6	21.2	24.9	28.6
10500	14.3	17.7	21.3	24.9	28.7
11000	14.4	17.8	21.3	25.0	28.8
11500	14.4	17.8	21.4	25.1	28.9
12000	14.5	17.9	21.5	25.2	28.9
13000	14.6	18.0	21.6	25.3	29.1
14000	14.7	18.1	21.7	25.4	29.2
15000	14.8	18.2	21.8	25.5	29.3
16000	14.9	18.3	21.9	25.6	29.4
17000	15.0	18.4	22.0	25.7	29.5
18000	15.1	18.5	22.1	25.8	29.6
19000	15.1	18.6	22.2	25.9	29.7
20000	15.2	18.7	22.3	26.0	29.8
21000	15.3	18.8	22.4	26.1	29.9
22000	15.4	18.8	22.4	26.1	29.9
23000	15.4	18.9	22.5	26.2	30.0
24000	15.5	19.0	22.6	26.3	30.1
25000	15.6	19.0	22.6	26.4	30.1
26000	15.6	19.1	22.7	26.4	30.2
27000	15.7	19.1	22.8	26.5	30.3
29000	15.8	19.3	22.9	26.6	30.4
32000	15.9	19.4	23.0	26.8	30.6
34000	16.0	19.5	23.1	26.9	30.7
36000	16.1	19.6	23.2	26.9	30.8
38000	16.2	19.7	23.3	27.0	30.8
40000	16.3	19.8	23.4	27.1	30.9
42000	16.3	19.8	23.5	27.2	31.0
44000	16.4	19.9	23.5	27.3	31.1
46000	16.5	20.0	23.6	27.3	31.2
50000	16.6	20.1	23.7	27.5	31.3
54000	16.7	20.2	23.9	27.6	31.4
58000	16.8	20.3	24.0	27.7	31.5
62000	16.9	20.4	24.1	27.8	31.7
66000	17.0	20.5	24.2	27.9	31.8
70000	17.1	20.6	24.3	28.0	31.9
75000	17.2	20.7	24.4	28.2	32.0
80000	17.3	20.8	24.5	28.3	32.1
85000	17.4	20.9	24.6	28.4	32.2
90000	17.5	21.0	24.7	28.5	32.3

Bioburden	10^{-2}	10^{-3}	10^{-4}	10^{-5}	10^{-6}
95000	17.6	21.1	24.8	28.5	32.4
100000	17.6	21.2	24.9	28.6	32.5
110000	17.8	21.3	25.0	28.8	32.6
120000	17.9	21.5	25.2	28.9	32.8
130000	18.0	21.6	25.3	29.1	32.9
140000	18.1	21.7	25.4	29.2	33.0
150000	18.2	21.8	25.5	29.3	33.1
160000	18.3	21.9	25.6	29.4	33.3
170000	18.4	22.0	25.7	29.5	33.4
180000	18.5	22.1	25.8	29.6	33.4
190000	18.6	22.2	25.9	29.7	33.5
200000	18.7	22.3	26.0	29.8	33.6
220000	18.8	22.4	26.1	29.9	33.8
240000	19.0	22.6	26.3	30.1	33.9
260000	19.1	22.7	26.4	30.2	34.1
280000	19.2	22.8	26.5	30.3	34.2
300000	19.3	22.9	26.6	30.4	34.3
320000	19.4	23.0	26.8	30.6	34.4
340000	19.5	23.1	26.9	30.7	34.5
360000	19.6	23.2	26.9	30.8	34.6
380000	19.7	23.3	27.0	30.8	34.7
400000	19.8	23.4	27.1	30.9	34.8
420000	19.8	23.5	27.2	31.0	34.9
440000	19.9	23.5	27.3	31.1	35.0
460000	20.0	23.6	27.3	31.2	35.0
480000	20.0	23.7	27.4	31.2	35.1
500000	20.1	23.7	27.5	31.3	35.2
540000	20.2	23.9	27.6	31.4	35.3
580000	20.3	24.0	27.7	31.5	35.4
620000	20.4	24.1	27.8	31.7	35.5
660000	20.5	24.2	27.9	31.8	35.6
700000	20.6	24.3	28.0	31.9	35.7
750000	20.7	24.4	28.2	32.0	35.9
800000	20.8	24.5	28.3	32.1	36.0
850000	20.9	24.6	28.4	32.2	36.1
900000	21.0	24.7	28.5	32.3	36.2
950000	21.1	24.8	28.5	32.4	36.3
1000000	21.2	24.9	28.6	32.5	36.3

Glossary

Absorbed dose: quantity of radiation energy imparted per unit mass of matter. The unit of absorbed dose is the gray (Gy), where 1 gray is equivalent to absorption of 1 joule per kilogram (= 100 rads).

Action level(s): established microbiological level(s) set by the user in the context of controlled environments. When action levels are exceeded, immediate follow-up is required and should trigger an investigation, and corrective action should be taken based on the investigation.

Acute systemic toxicity: estimates the harmful effects of either single or multiple exposures to test materials and/or extracts in an animal model during a period of less than 24 hours.

Aerobic organisms: microorganisms that utilize oxygen as the final electron acceptor during metabolism and which will only grow in the presence of oxygen.

Alert level(s): established microbiological level(s) set by the user for controlled environments, giving early warning of a potential drift from normal conditions. When alert levels are exceeded, an investigation should be conducted to ensure that the process and/or environment are under control.

Anaerobic organisms: microorganisms that do not utilize oxygen as the final electron acceptor during metabolism and which will only grow in the absence of oxygen.

Augmentation: action taken to increase the sterilization dose based upon the results obtained from a sterilization dose audit.

Average beam current: time-averaged current produced by an electron beam generator.

Bacteriostasis/fungistasis test: test performed with selected microorganisms to demonstrate the presence of substances that inhibit the multiplication of these microorganisms.

Batch: defined quantity of bulk, intermediate, or finished product that is intended or purported to be uniform in character and quality, and which has been produced during a defined cycle of manufacture.

Batch-type irradiator: irradiator in which the irradiation containers are introduced or removed while the radioactive source is in the storage room.

Beam current: a measure of the number of electrons exiting an accelerator each second.

Beam energy: the kinetic energy carried by each particle in an electron beam.

Bioburden: population of viable microorganisms on raw material, a component, a finished product, and/or a package just prior to sterilization.

Bioburden estimate: value established for the number of microorganisms comprising the bioburden by applying to a viable count or presterilization counts a factor compensating for the recovery efficiency.

Bremsstrahlung: broad spectrum electromagnetic radiation emitted when an energetic electron is influenced by a strong magnetic or electric field, such as that in the vicinity of an atomic nucleus.

Bulk density: mass of product and all associated packaging in the irradiation container divided by the volume determined by the dimensions of the outermost packaging.

Calibration: comparison of a measurement system or device of unknown accuracy to a measurement system or device of known accuracy (traceable to national standards) to detect, correlate, report, or eliminate by adjustment, any variation from the required performance limits of the unverified measurement system or device.

Carcinogenesis bioassay: the determination of the tumorogenic potential of test materials and/or extracts from either single or multiple exposures, over a period of the total life (e.g., 2 years for rat, 18 months for mouse, or 7 years for dog).

Certification: documented reviews and approval process carried out as a final step in the validation program to permit product release.

Chronic toxicity: the determination of harmful effects from multiple exposures to test materials and/or extracts during a period of 10% to the total life of the test animal (e.g., over 90 days in rats).

Cleanroom: a room in which the number concentration of airborne particles is controlled, and which is constructed and used in a manner to minimize the introduction, generation, and retention of particles inside the room and in which other relevant parameters, e.g., temperature, humidity, and pressure, are controlled, if necessary.

Colony-forming unit (cfu): visible growth of microorganisms arising from a single cell or multiple cells.

Commissioning (installation qualification): obtaining and documenting evidence that equipment has been provided and installed in accordance with its specifications and that it functions within predetermined limits when operated in accordance with operational instructions (*see also* **validation**).

Contact plate: contact device containing agar where the container is a rigid dish.

Continuous-type irradiator: irradiator that can be loaded and unloaded with product while the source is in the processing mode.

Converter: target for high-energy electron beams, generally of high atomic number, in which X-rays are produced by radioactive energy losses of the incident beam.

Corrective action: action(s) to be taken when the results of monitoring biocontamination indicate a loss of control or when action levels are exceeded.

Culture conditions: stated combination of conditions, including the growth medium with the period and temperature of incubation, used to promote growth and multiplication of microorganisms.

Curie: a quantity of radioactive isotope in which 37 billion nuclear transformations take place per second.

Cytotoxicity: test that determines, with the use of cell culture techniques, the lysis of cells, the inhibition of growth, and other toxic effects on cells caused by test materials and/or extracts.

D_{10}-**value (decimal reduction value):** dose (expressed in kGy) required to achieve inactivation of 90% of a population of the test organisms under stated exposure conditions where it is assumed that the death of microorganisms follows first order kinetics.

Dose uniformity ratio: the ratio of the maximum dose divided by the minimum dose.

Dosimeter: device or system having a reproducible, measurable response to radiation, which can be used to measure the absorbed dose in a given material.

Dosimetry system: system used for determining absorbed dose, consisting of dosimeters, and measuring instrumentation and procedures for the system's use.

Electron: a small, negatively charged subatomic particle.

Electron beam: continuous or pulsed stream of high energy electrons.

Electron energy: kinetic energy of the electrons in the electron beam.

Environmental controls: controls established in product manufacturing areas to control bioburden.

Environmental monitoring program: defined documented program that describes the routine particulate and microbiological testing to be performed in manufacturing areas and that includes a corrective action plan when action levels are exceeded.

Facultative organisms: microorganisms capable of aerobic and anaerobic metabolism.

False negative: test results interpreted as no growth, either where growth was present but not detected, or where viable microorganisms failed to grow.

False positive: result of a test of sterility where turbidity is interpreted as growth arising from the sample tested, when the growth resulted from extraneous microbial contamination or the turbidity arose from an interaction between the sample and the test medium.

Fractional positive: quotient with the number of positive sterility tests in the numerator and the number of samples in the denominator.

Gamma ray: short wavelength electromagnetic radiation (photons) emitted from radioactive substances in the process of nuclear transition.

Genotoxicity: *see* **mutagenicity**.

Growth promotion test: test performed to demonstrate that a given medium will support microbial growth.

Half-life: the time required for a radioactive isotope to decay to half its original curie content.

Hemocompatibility: test that evaluates any effects of blood-contacting materials on hemolysis, thrombosis, plasma proteins, enzymes, and the formed elements using an animal model.

Hemolysis: test that determines the degree of red blood cell lysis and the separation of hemoglobin caused by test materials and/or extracts from the materials *in vitro*.

Implantation tests: tests that evaluate local toxic effects on living tissue, at both the gross level and microscopic level, to a sample material that is surgically implanted into an appropriate animal implant site or tissue for 7–90 days.

Inactivation: loss of the ability of microorganisms to germinate, outgrow, and/or multiply under specified culture conditions.

Incremental dose: dose within a series applied to a number of product units or portions thereof and used in dose setting methods to establish or confirm the sterilization dose.

Irradiator: assembly that permits safe and reliable sterilization processing, including the source of the radiation, conveyor and source mechanisms, safety devices, and shield.

Irradiator operator: company of body responsible for delivery of a specified dose to health care products.

Irritation: test that estimates the irritation and sensitization potential of test materials and their extracts, using appropriate site or implant tissue such as skin and mucous membrane in an animal model and/or human.

Medical device: any instrument, apparatus, appliance, material, or other article, whether used alone or in combination, including the software necessary for its proper application intended by the manufacturer to be used for human beings for the following purposes:

- diagnosis, prevention, monitoring, treatment, or alleviation of disease
- diagnosis, monitoring, treatment, alleviation of, or compensation for an injury or handicap
- investigation, replacement, or modification of the anatomy or of a physiological process
- control of conception

It does not achieve its principal intended action in or on the human body by pharmacological, immunological or metabolic means, but may be assisted in its function by such means.

Microbial barrier: ability to prevent the ingress of microorganisms.

Microbicidal effectiveness: demonstrated lethal action of the sterilizing agent against a representative range of microorganisms.

Microbiological quantity: product bioburden and microbial resistance to radiation.

Microorganism: any one-celled unit of sporangia and non-sporangia bacteria, viruses, fungi, and protozoa.

Mutagenicity (genotoxicity): the application of mammalian or non-mammalian cell culture techniques for the determination of gene mutations, changes in chromosome structure and number, and other DNA or gene tonicities caused by test materials and/or extracts from materials.

National standard: standard recognized by an official national decision as basis for fixing the value, in a country, of all other standards of the quantity concerned.

Performance qualification: obtaining and documenting evidence that the equipment as commissioned will produce acceptable product when operated in accordance with the process specification (*see also* **validation**).

Photon: a particle that has no mass or charge and is the basic unit of electromagnetic energy.

Primary standard dosimeter: dosimeter, of the highest metrological quality, established and maintained as an absorbed dose standard by a national or international standards organization.

Process development: documented program of studies, which is performed in order to define the sterilization process based upon the product/packaging/loading pattern and/or equipment limitations.

Process interruption: intentional or unintentional stoppage of the irradiation processing.

Process parameter: specified value for a process variable.

Process qualification: obtaining and documenting evidence that the sterilization process will produce acceptable health care products.

Process variable: condition within a sterilization process in which changes alter the microbicidal effectiveness of the process.

Product: generic term used to describe raw materials, intermediate products, subassemblies, and finished medical devices.

Product compatibility: ability of the sterilization process to achieve the intended results without detrimental effect to the product.

Product families: group of products with common characteristics and similar microbiological characteristics that require the same minimum sterilization dose.

Product qualification: obtaining and documenting evidence that the health care product will be acceptable for its intended use after exposure to radiation.

Product unit: health care product, collection of products or components within a primary package.

Recovery efficiency: measure of the ability of a specified technique to remove microorganisms from product.

Reference load: specified sterilization load made up to represent the most difficult combination of products to be sterilized.

Revalidation: repetition of part of validation to confirm the continued acceptability of a specified process.

Routine dosimeter: dosimeter calibrated against a primary reference or transfer standard dosimeter and used for routine dosimetry measurement.

Sample item portion (SIP): defined portion of a health care product unit that is tested.

Sampling plan: sample size or sizes to be used and associated acceptance criteria.

Source activity: quantity of the radionucleotide ^{60}Co or ^{137}Cs measured in becquerels of curies (1 curie $= 3.7 \times 10^{10}$ becquerels, where 1 becquerel $= 1$ disintegration per second).

Spore log reduction (SLR): the lethality observed in a full or fractional sterilization cycle. SLR can be calculated as the log of the initial population minus the log of the final population.

$$\text{SLR} = \log (N_o) - \log N_f$$

If there are no survivors, the true SLR cannot be calculated. If one positive is assumed for the purposes of calculation, the SLR should be reported as "greater than."

Standard distribution of resistance (SDR): a hypothetical distribution (based on measurements of the radiation resistances of selected microbial isolates) comprising a series of increasing D_{10} values and associated probabilities of occurrence.

Sterile: free from viable microorganisms (*see also* **sterilization**).

Sterility: state of being free from viable microorganisms (*see also* **sterilization**). *Note:* in practice, no such absolute statement regarding the absence of microorganisms can be proven.

Sterility assurance level (SAL): probability of a viable microorganism being present on a product unit after sterilization. SAL is normally expressed as 10^{-n}.

Sterility test: test performed to determine if viable microorganisms are present.

Sterilization: validated process used to render a product free of all forms of viable microorganisms. *Note:* In a sterilization process, the nature of microbial death is described by an exponential function. Therefore, the presence of viable microorganisms on any individual item can be expressed in terms of probability. While this probability may be reduced to a very low number, it can never be reduced to zero. The probability can be expressed as a sterility assurance level (SAL).

Sterilization dose audit: action taken to detect whether or not a change in sterilization dose is needed.

Sterilization load: goods that are to be or have been sterilized simultaneously in the same sterilization chamber. *Note:* the sterilization load may include more than one manufacturing batch or lot.

Sterilization process: all treatments that are required to accomplish sterilization to include preconditioning (if used), the sterilization cycle, and aeration.

Surface density: density of a columnar section through product within its outermost packaging or through the irradiation container, in the direction of the electron beam, expressed as a ratio against the surface area of the section at a position where the ratio takes its highest value.

Survival-kill window: extent of exposure to a sterilization process under defined conditions when there is a transition from all biological indicators showing growth (survival exposure) to all biological indicators showing no growth (kill exposure).

Survivor curve: graphical representation of inactivation against increasing exposure to stated conditions.

Swabbing: sampling of viable particles by stroking a defined surface area with a swab that has been premoistened with an appropriate extraction fluid (eluent).

Test of sterility: test performed to establish the presence or absence of viable microorganisms on product units (or portions thereof) when subjected to defined culture conditions.

Timer setting: interval of time selected for the irradiation container to spend at each position within the irradiator. It controls the duration of radiation exposure.

Traceability: the property of a result of a measurement whereby it can be related to appropriate standards, generally international and national standards, through an unbroken chain of comparisons.

Transfer standard dosimeter: dosimeter, often a reference standard dosimeter, intended for transport between different locations for use as an intermediary to compare absorbed dose measurements.

VD_{max}: maximal acceptable verification dose for a given bioburden and verification sample size.

Validation: documented procedure for obtaining, recording, and interpreting the results needed to show that a process will consistently yield a product complying with predetermined specifications. *Note:* validation is considered a total process that consists of commissioning and performance qualification. The relationship between these terms is illustrated above.

Verification dose ($D**$ kGy): a dose of radiation estimated to produce an SAL of 10^{-2} for a product unit or portion thereof, and used in dose setting methods to establish or confirm the sterilization dose.

Viable count: number of microorganisms estimated by growth of discrete colonies under the stated culture conditions.

X-rays: short wavelength electromagnetic radiation emitted by high-energy electrons when they are accelerated, decelerated, or deflected by strong electric or magnetic fields.

Bibliography

American Society for Testing and Materials, F1980-99el, *Standard Guide for Accelerated Aging of Sterile Medical Device Packages*, ASTM, West Conshohocken, PA, 2000.

Association for the Advancement of Medical Instrumentation, ANSI/AAMI/ISO 11137, *Sterilization of health care products—Requirements for validation and routine control—Radiation sterilization*, AAMI, Arlington VA, 1995.

Association for the Advancement of Medical Instrumentation, AAMI TIR 15843, *Sterilization of health care products—Radiant sterilization—Product families, sampling plans for verification dose experiments and sterilization dose audits, and frequency of sterilization dose audits*, AAMI, Arlington, VA, 1999.

Association for the Advancement of Medical Instrumentation, AAMI TIR 15844, *Sterilization of health care products—Radiation sterilization—Selection of a sterilization dose for a single production batch*, AAMI, Arlington, VA, 1998.

Association for the Advancement of Medical Instrumentation, AAMI TIR 17, *Radiation sterilization—Material qualification*, AAMI, Arlington, VA, 1998.

Association for the Advancement of Medical Instrumentation, AAMI/CD-1 TIR, *Sterilization of health care products—Radiation sterilization—Substantiation of 25 kGy as a sterilization dose*, AAMI draft, 2000.

Association for the Advancement of Medical Instrumentation, ANSI/AAMI/ISO 11737-1: 1995, *Sterilization of medical devices—Microbiological methods—Part 1: Estimation of the population of microorganisms on product*, AAMI, Arlington, VA, 1995.

Association for the Advancement of Medical Instrumentation, ANSI/AAMI/ISO 11737-2:1998, *Sterilization of medical devices—Microbiological methods—Part 2: Test of sterility performed in the validation of a sterilization process*, AAMI, Arlington, VA, 1998.

Association for the Advancement of Medical Instrumentation, ISO/CD 11737-3, *Sterilization of medical devices—Microbiological methods—Part 3: Guidance on the evaluation and interpretation of bioburden data*, AAMI draft, Arlington, VA, 2000.

Association for the Advancement of Medical Instrumentation, ANSI/AAMI/ISO 10993-1: 1995, *Biological evaluation of medical devices—Part 1: Guidance on selection of tests*, AAMI, Arlington, VA.

Association for the Advancement of Medical Instrumentation, ANSI/AAMI/ISO 10993-5, *Biological evaluation of medical devices—Tests for cytotoxicity,* in vitro *methods,* AAMI, Arlington, VA, 1993.

Association for the Advancement of Medical Instrumentation, AAMI Draft ST 67, *Sterilization of medical devices—Requirements for products labeled "Sterile,"* AAMI, Arlington, VA.

Bernard, John W., "E-Beam Processing in the Medial Device Industry," *Med. Dev. Tech.,* June, 1991.

Bryans, Trabue, "Using Bioburden Spikes in Radiation Dose-Setting," *The Validation Consultant,* Vol. 3 No. 1, January, 1996.

Barcan, Donald S., "The Effects of Radiation Sterilization on Package Seal Strength," *Med. Dev. & Diag. Ind.,* November, 1994.

Booth, Anne F., ed., *Sterilization of Medical Devices,* InterPharm Press, Denver, CO, 1999.

Booth, Anne and Gibson, James Jr., "Custom Kits: An Opportunity for Radiation Sterilization?" Presentation at *4th Nordion Gamma Processing Seminar,* May, 1991.

EN 552: *Sterilization of medical devices—Validation and routine control of sterilization by irradiation,* 1994.

EN 556: *Sterilization of medical devices—Requirements for medical devices to be labeled sterile.*

Farrell, J. Paul and Hemmerich, Karl J., "Selecting a Radiation Sterilization Method," *Med. Dev. & Diag. Ind.,* August, 1995.

FDA, *Guideline on Validation of the Limulus Amebocyte Lysate Test as an End-Product Endotoxin Test for Human and Animal Parenteral Drugs, Biological Products and Medical Devices,* December, 1987.

Hansen, Joyce and Whitby, James, "Gamma Radiation Sterilization Practice in the U.S. Device Industry," *Med. Dev. & Diag. Ind.,* July, 1994.

Hansen, Joyce, Shaffer, Harry, Bryans, Trabue, Reger, John and Duda, Denise, "Investigating AAMI Radiation Audit Results," *Med. Dev. & Diag. Ind.,* May, 1994.

Hemmerich, Karl J., "General Aging Theory and Simplified Protocol for Accelerated Aging of Medical Devices," *Med. Plastics and Biomat.,* July/August, 1998.

Herring, C., "Dose Audit Failures and Dose Augmentation," *Radiat. Phys. Chem.,* 54, 1999.

Hoxey, E. V., "Validation of Methods for Bioburden Estimation," *Sterilization of Medical Products,* Vol. VI, Proceedings of the International Kilmer Conference, Brussels, Belgium, 1993.

International Atomic Energy Agency, *Guidelines for Industrial Sterilization of Disposable Medical Products, Co^{60} Gamma Radiation.* TEC DOC-539. Vienna: IAEA, 1990.

Kowalski, John B., Aoshuang, Yan and Tallentire, Alan, "Radiation Sterilization—Evaluation of an Improved Method of Substantiation of 25 kGy," *Radiat., Phys. Chem.,* 54, 1999.

Kowalski, John B. and Tallentire, Alan, "Substantiation of 25 kGy as a Sterilization Dose: A Rational Approach to Establishing Verification Dose," *Radiat. Phys. Chem.* 54, 1999.

Nolan, P. J., "Accelerated Aging of Medical Packages," *FDA Reg. & Qual. Advisor,* Vol. 6, No. 4, February, 1999.

Phillips, George W., Taylor, Wayne A., Sargent, Harold E. and Hansen, Joyce M., "Reducing Sample Sizes of AAMI Gamma Radiation Sterilization Verification Experiments and Dose Audits," *Quality Engineering,* 8(3), 1996.

Reid, Brain D. and Fairand, Barry P., "Gamma Radiation Sterilization of Pharmaceuticals," *Sterilization of Drugs and Devices,* Nordhauser and Olsen, eds., Interpharm Press, Buffalo Grove, IL, 1998.

Saylor, M. C. and Herring, C. M., "Dose Setting, Process Control and U.S. Regulatory Compliance," Presentation at *4th Nordion Gamma Processing Seminar,* May 1991.

Saunders, Chris, Lucht, Lisa and McDougall, Tom, "Radiant Effects on Microorganisms and Polymers for Medical Products," *Med. Dev. & Diag. Ind.,* May, 1993.

Stumbo, C. R., Murphy, J. R. and Cockran, J., "Nature of Thermal Death Time Curves for P.A. 3676 and *Clostridium botulinum,*" *Food Tech.,* 4, 1950.

Tallentire, Alan, "Radiation Dose Setting/Substantiation Methods: Have We Got It Right?" *Sterilization of Medical Products,* Vol. VII, Morrissey and Kowalski, eds., Polyscience Publications Inc., Champlain, NY, 1998.

Williams, John, "Weighing the Choices in Radiation Sterilization: Electron-Beam and Gamma," *Med. Dev. & Diag. Ind.,* March, 1995.

Whitby, J. L., "Radiation Resistance of Microorganisms Comprising the Bioburden of Operating Room Packs," *Radiat. Phys. Chem.,* 14, 1979.

T - #0586 - 101024 - C0 - 222/150/9 - PB - 9781138561939 - Gloss Lamination